PRAISE FOR

EAT LESS WATER

"Water is life; a fundamental human right. The movement to protect our water resources is here. We must all participate if we are to save Mother Earth. *Eat Less Water* is an impassioned call to action. Read, learn, and act. Florencia Ramirez shows us how."

—DOLORES HUERTA

Co-Founder of the United Farm Workers, Presidential Medal of Freedom Recipient, and President of the Dolores Huerta Foundation

"*Eat Less Water* is as clever as its title. It's a thoughtful book complete with recipes that are as good for your taste buds as they are for the planet. Read it and learn. Read it and eat. Read it as a reminder that our world's most precious resource is in jeopardy—and yet we can do something about it. Read it to find out how."

—THOMAS M. KOSTIGEN

New York Times bestselling author of *The Green Book*

"*Eat Less Water* is an informative, loving tribute to the source from which all life springs. Through explorations of foods ranging from pasta to wine, Florencia Ramirez reveals how cultivation and consumption impact global water usage, sharing insights on how we, the eaters, can support a less-resource intensive practices in food and agriculture that is not only sustainable but delicious."

—SIMRAN SETHI

author of *Bread, Wine, Chocolate: The Slow Loss of Foods We Love*

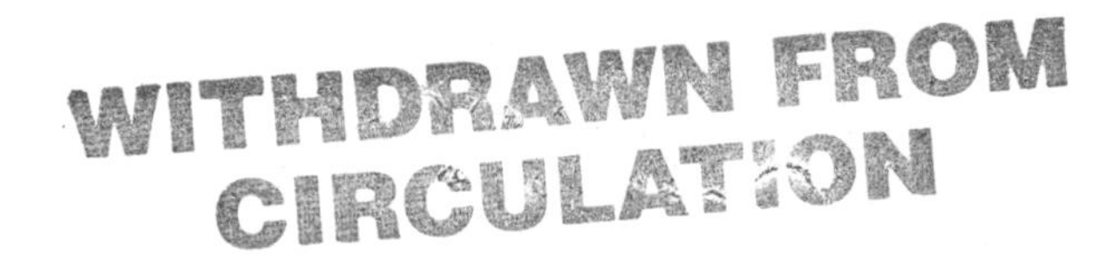

EAT LESS WATER

Florencia Ramirez

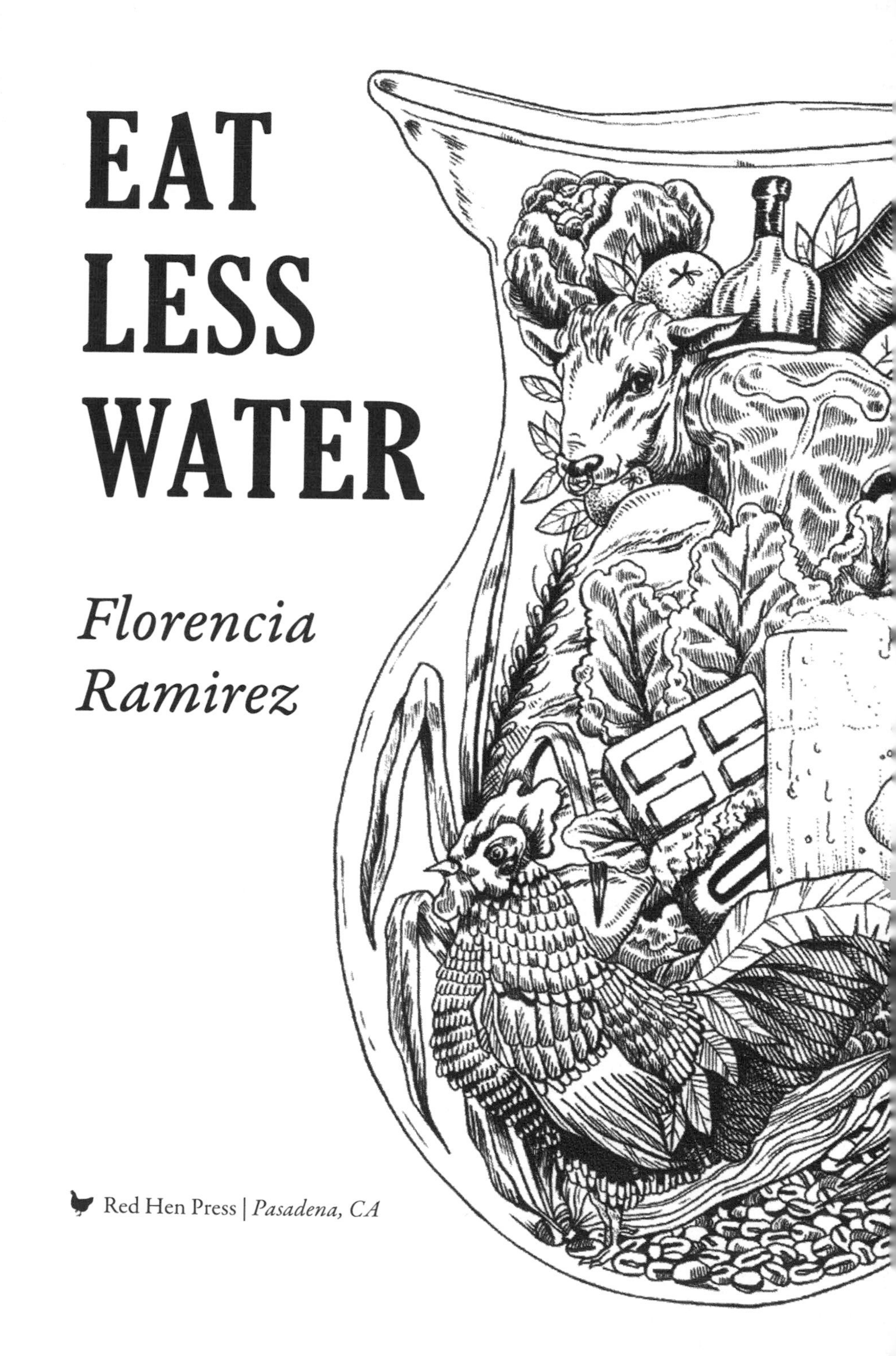

Red Hen Press | *Pasadena, CA*

Book design by Selena Trager

Names: Ramirez, Florencia, author.
Title: Eat less water / Florencia Ramirez.
Description: Pasadena, CA : Red Hen Press, [2017]
Identifiers: LCCN 2017011414 | ISBN 9781597090391 (pbk. : alk. paper) | ISBN 9781597095143 (ebook)
Subjects: LCSH: Cooking. | Water conservation. | Water consumption. | Water in agriculture. | Drinking water. | LCGFT: Cookbooks.
Classification: LCC TX714 .R354 2017 | DDC 641.5—dc23
LC record available at https://lccn.loc.gov/2017011414

The National Endowment for the Arts, the Los Angeles County Arts Commission, the Dwight Stuart Youth Fund, the Max Factor Family Foundation, the Pasadena Tournament of Roses Foundation, the Pasadena Arts & Culture Commission and the City of Pasadena Cultural Affairs Division, the City of Los Angeles Department of Cultural Affairs, the Audrey & Sydney Irmas Charitable Foundation, Sony Pictures Entertainment, Amazon Literary Partnership, and the Sherwood Foundation partially support Red Hen Press.

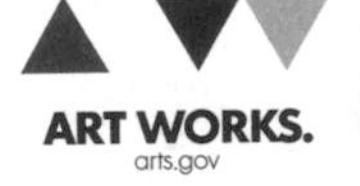

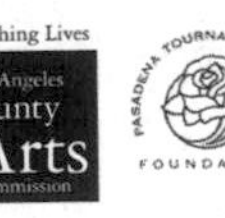

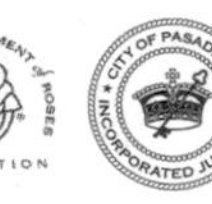

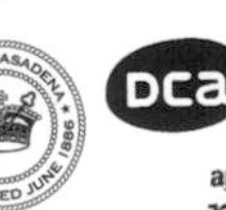

DCA DEPARTMENT OF CULTURAL AFFAIRS
City of Los Angeles

amazon literary partnership

First Edition
Published by Red Hen Press
www.redhen.org

For Michael,

what's mine is yours *para siempre*

CONTENTS

Prologue: Drop of Water 1

Introduction: Food & Water 3

1. Wheat & Water 17

2. Rice & Water 27

3. Produce & Water 44

4. Aquaponics & Water 57

5. Seafood & Water 66

6. Soy, Corn & Water 80

7. Eggs & Water 88

8. Chicken & Water 98

9. Dairy & Water 107

10. Meat & Water 124

11. Chocolate & Water 143

12. Coffee & Water 159

13. Wine & Water 170

14. Tequila & Water 183

15. Beer & Water 190

16. Gardens & Water 205

Epilogue: The Solution Is in the Kitchen...... 221

Index of Recipes 229

Eat Less Water

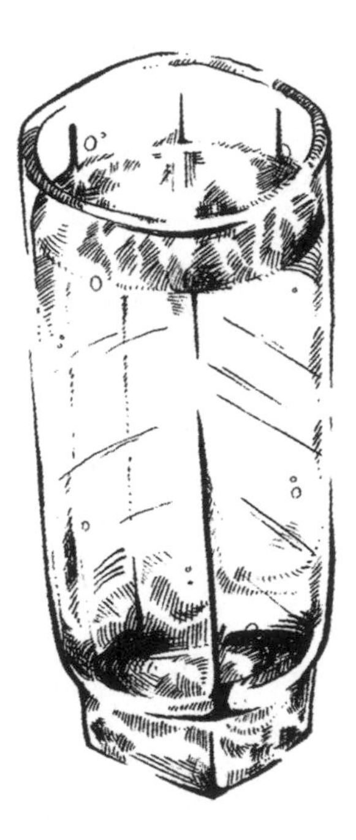

PROLOGUE

Drop of Water

DROPS OF WATER saved my father's life.

In the sweltering days following my father's birth, he just lay there. He did not cry. He refused milk.

On the fourth day, my grandmother sent her daughter to borrow a small table from the neighbor's chicken coop. They would need something to put his tiny body on, for the family viewing. My grandmother knew the signs of a dying baby. She'd given birth to eleven children. Only seven survived.

My father's sister came back with the table, but she refused to give up on her newborn brother. There had to be a doctor who would examine a baby for free. She ran through the heat of the Mexican summer to the town center and began knocking on doors.

Someone knew a doctor, but he was busy with other patients. When he listened to her, this little girl desperate about her baby brother, the physician agreed to make a house call the next day.

That night, a strong wind blew through the open window of the bedroom where my father lay. The gust startled my grandfather awake. He threw himself over my father's listless body to shield him against what my grandfather always described as an otherworldly chill. A cold hand pressed down on his back. He believed it was the hand of *La Muerte*, Death.

The cold wind retreated as suddenly as it arrived. My father was still alive, just barely.

The doctor arrived the next morning. After a quick examination, he knew what was wrong. He prescribed *gotitas de agua*. Drops of water on the baby's lips.

Within days, my father's condition slowly improved. He suffered from dehydration. His sister, my *tia* Antonia, returned the table to the neighbors, back to the chicken coop where it belonged.

When I told this story to my friends at school, I always made sure to emphasize the part about Death paying a visit only to leave empty-handed.

~

"Did you know one drop of water holds all the fresh water in the world?" a retired park ranger asked me at my booth where I sold water conservation products during an Earth Day event.

"How so?"

"If we poured all the water on our planet, both salt water and fresh water, in a gallon bucket, the proportion of water available to shower, water our lawns, drink, and grow food is one single drop."

We live on a water planet. The Earth is two-thirds water, and 97.5 percent of that is salt water. Of the 2.5 percent fresh water, 69.5 percent of that is frozen. Another 30.1 percent hides in deep aquifers. The remaining 0.4 percent—a drop in a bucket—sustains all the life on this planet.

Now when I tell my father's story to my own children, I emphasize the power of a single drop of water.

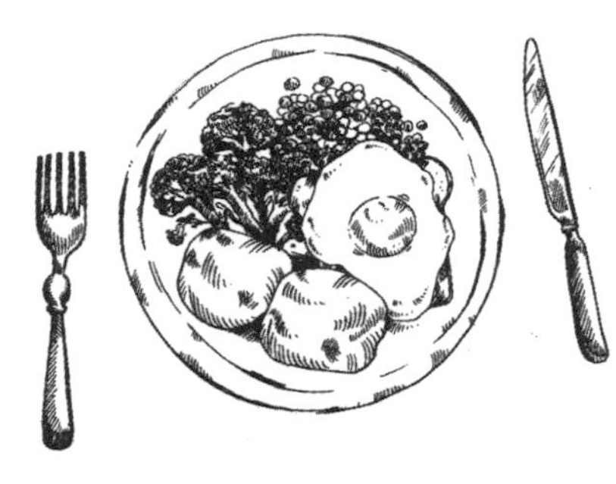

INTRODUCTION
Food & Water

THE MOST FAR-REACHING, effective strategy to save water is to eat less of it. Realizing this is what led me to start reading labels and replacing our family's favorite brands of conventionally raised food with organic alternatives. The transition went largely unnoticed by my kids until my changes in the menu reached the cereal shelf in the kitchen pantry.

"Where's my cornflakes?" my seven-year-old daughter Isabella demanded.

"I got us some new cereals to try." I showed her the choices.

"What's wrong with the kind we always eat?"

"These are better for water," I answered, pointing to the USDA organic seal.

"*Water*? It's not like cornflakes come soggy," she griped.

"Food grown without chemicals saves fresh water more than any other water-saving strategy."

Now I had her confused, an improvement over defiant. She'd heard the story about the drops of water saving my father's life, and she'd watched my growing passion to conserve water take over the house. It had led to my starting up a small business distributing shower timers.

Isabella, as the eldest of three, had joined me at Earth Day events and trade shows. She helped me cover portable tables with blue cloth and stack star- and duck-shaped shower timers in neat displays. She had listened to me rattle off statistics. "You can save 2,500 gallons of water in one year," I told people. Together we sold 80,000 shower timers.

"Isn't taking shorter showers enough?" Isabella moaned, still yearning for her old cornflakes.

I explained that my focus on the shower had been misguided. The same amount of water saved over the course of a year in the bathroom can be saved in a *week* in the kitchen, because seven out of every ten gallons of water is used for food production. I'd been focusing on the wrong room of the house.

A pound of beef has a "virtual water footprint" of 1,851 gallons. Virtual water isn't directly visible in food products but the concept captures the total amount of water required to produce food. The virtual water footprint of beef represents not just the water a cow drinks, but also the water used to grow all the grain or grass consumed by the average cow over its lifetime. A loaf of bread has a virtual water footprint of 425 gallons, representing the water required to grow and harvest the grain.[1]

The United Nations reports each American eats between 530 and 1,300 gallons of virtual water every day. The water footprint of the United States is more than twice that of any other nation.

Of course, the water required to grow food doesn't disappear. Water's ability to change state from solid, liquid, and gas allows for its endless movement around our planet. When water is drawn from underground aquifers to irrigate crops, the water isn't gone, but through evaporation and runoff, as much as 50 percent of the water pumped to the surface moves on.[2] When the water moves away faster than it gets replaced, farmland eventually becomes parched and deserts spread. That's

1. These are simplified descriptions of complex algorithms researchers use to calculate water footprints. Find a wealth of studies on water footprint at http://www.waterfootprint.org.

2. See the State of Washington Department of Ecology website at http://www.ecy.wa.gov/programs/wr/ws/wtrcnsv.html.

happening now, leaving more than one billion people and counting without sufficient water.

~

A Facebook friend posted a furious report about her neighbor, describing him as "selfish" and "irresponsible." His offense? He watered his rose bushes during a drought. Many of the thirty-two responses urged her to report him to the city. She posted she already had.

I didn't reply or hit the "like" button. While I'm glad awareness of the need to conserve water is catching on with the public, sometimes people's attempts to do something, anything, can be exasperating. There is no lasting effect on the planet to turning your neighbor in for watering his roses or, God forbid, hosing down his driveway, apart from upsetting your particular neighborhood.

During each drought period, there is a heightened awareness of water. Articles printed in newspapers and magazines report low reservoir levels, dry wells, and unplanted fields blowing away. From Texas to Tennessee, electric road signs and billboards read SEVERE DROUGHT and SAVE WATER, and we become unofficially deputized as water cops, vigilantes deployed to report the neighbor watering his rose bush.

Then when the drought is declared over, it's the news stories that dry up and blow away. Billboards are replaced, and the conversation moves on to the next crisis. But we remain in the same predicament. Half the world population will experience freshwater shortages, referred to as "water scarcity" events, by 2030.[3] Water scarcity is expected to result in the deaths of millions and an unprecedented rise in military conflicts. Of all the crises coming to a head, water scarcity is the least understood.

---

3. See the United Nations Department of Economic and Social Affairs (UNDESA) website. It includes links to UN publications available for free download on areas of water scarcity, climate change and food security. http://www.un.org/waterforlifedecade/scarcity.shtml.

Supply and quality are the two leading causes of water scarcity, according to the United Nations. I don't need to travel far from my home to understand why.

Thousands of agricultural acres grow forty-six different crops year-round in my hometown. Agriculture brought my family to Oxnard, California, three generations ago. One set of grandparents worked in the fields as farm workers. The other set worked in a sugar beet packing house.

Oxnard's breeze is fragrant with crisp celery some months, sweet strawberries in others. Our crops are exported worldwide: plump strawberries enjoyed with tea at Wimbledon and served for dessert in Japan. Sprinkler heads spray groundwater to keep these crops verdant. Irrigation replaces natural rain in this part of California, and gives the impression of abundant supply—but this is an illusion.

Water is drawn from underground quicker than rainfall and seepage can naturally replace it. Groundwater levels in my coastal town drop by 300,000 acre-feet or ninety-eight billion gallons each year, enough water to fill nearly 150,000 Olympic-size pools. And this is in non-drought years. The deficit increases more during dry years.[4]

The lowered water table is out of view, but the missing water is evident in the disappearing rivers and streams in the region; those not paved over in cement have wilted to trickles or trails of dust. Born and raised in California, I once thought all farms were irrigated. In fact, 90 percent of the world's food is grown exclusively with natural rain. The problem is farms that use irrigation consume 70 percent of our planet's finite supply of freshwater resources.[5] And as the global climate warms,

4. Dennis Dimick, "If You Think the Water Crisis Can't Get Worse, Wait Until the Aquifers Are Drained," *National Geographic*, August 21, 2014, http://news.nationalgeographic.com/news/2014/08/140819-groundwater-california-drought-aquifers-hidden-crisis. During droughts, groundwater use increases. In California groundwater use totals increase from 40 percent to 60 percent.

5. "Statistics," UN Water, August 26, 2013, http://www.unwater.org/water-facts/water-food-and-energy/.

farmland once rain-fed will transition to irrigated land. Irrigated farms grow up to double the food of rain-fed farms, but use three times the water.[6] Can we afford to use three times the water? If not, how will we feed two billion more people on the planet by 2030?

The United States Geological Service (USGS) estimates groundwater provides 40 percent of our nation's public water supply. States like Florida, New Mexico, and Idaho are far above the average. Idaho almost exclusively uses groundwater (96 percent), followed by Florida (93 percent) and Mississippi (92 percent).[7] During droughts, the pumping rate jumps. Throughout dry years California draws 20 percent more groundwater. Even with regulation to take effect in 2040 in California, water tables will keep falling, leaving dry wells across the nation.

One of the world's largest aquifers, the Ogallala, stretching under eight states, dropped by over 160 feet in some areas according to the USGS, 95 percent of finite groundwater supplies pumped for irrigation. In every state, groundwater is treated as a *renewable* resource. But groundwater is finite. Although rain is always returning water to the ground, renewing an entire depleted aquifer can occur only very slowly, over years, decades, and millennia.

The shrinking water table led water managers in my town to seek solutions to meet the demand. One proposed solution is a $300 million state-of-the-art desalination and water treatment facility. The water is treated using a dozen chemicals to scrub away seawater salts. Brine laced with heavy metals from corrosion of pipes is discharged into the Pacific Ocean.[8] To pay for the energy-intensive process once the facility is com-

6. Fred Pearce, *When the Rivers Run Dry: Water—The Defining Crisis of the Twenty-First Century* (Boston: Beacon Press, 2007).
7. William M. Alley, Thomas E. Reilly, and O. Lehn Franke, "Sustainability of Ground-Water Resources," US Geological Survey, https://pubs.usgs.gov/circ/circ1186/html/intro.html.
8. Sabine Lattemann and Thomas Höpner, "Environmental Impact and Impact Assessment of Seawater Desalination," *Desalination: The International Journal on the Science and Technology of Desalting and Water Purification* 152, no. 1–3 (2003): 133–40.

pleted, consumers' water bills will increase, as desalination is three times more costly than pumping from aquifers.

"What's the light for?" asked my son Joaquin on a drive home from piano class. A spotlight flooded rows of strawberries, providing light for a tractor driver spraying pesticides. The night gave a typical sight an eerie quality. The light illuminated the thick chemical mist as it rose from the ground like steam.

The driver wore the required protective suit covering every inch of his body; his nose and mouth were covered with a surgical mask.

"Shouldn't he be wearing a gas mask?" asked Joaquin.

He was right. We think of serious protective gear as essential when dealing with contagious viruses or radioactive cleanups, but for workers growing the food we eat? The thought sends a shiver down the spine.

My proximity to conventional cropland in part influenced the decision to institute the "organic when available" policy my eldest daughter initially resisted when I replaced her cornflakes.

In 2011, 144 million gallons of chemical pesticides were sprayed onto cropland in the United States. Pesticides are applied as droplets, each lighter than dust.[9] The mist scatters and drifts, settles on surface water, and then leaches into water tables. The USGS tested 1,412 shallow wells in agricultural areas and found the presence of one or more pesticide products in 60 percent. The same study found nitrates in all the wells, with 21 percent at or higher than the US Environmental Protection Agency's (EPA) Maximum Contaminant Level.

NO DUMPING, DRAINS TO OCEAN, reads a sign near a storm ditch at the edge of a strawberry field. Twenty yards behind the sign loom

9. Over 17,000 pesticide products are registered in the United States containing 800 active ingredients. The EPA registers pesticides based on test results provided by the registrant, the producer of the chemical product. Toxicology testing on laboratory animals is required for each single active ingredient even though most formulas are a combination of substances.

liquid storage tanks of pesticides and fertilizers awaiting application to the surrounding fields.

Water contaminated with fertilizer runoff from fields and nutrients from animal feedlots are the largest polluter of rivers and groundwater. Forty percent of America's rivers and 46 percent of our lakes are too polluted with nitrates to support aquatic life according to the EPA. Over 1.65 trillion tons of nitrogen fed by the tributaries of thirty-six states pollutes the Mississippi River alone.[10]

Elevated nutrients in the water spur plant growth known as algal bloom. When in bloom, these plants are toxic to humans and fatal to animals. When the plant decomposes, it results in areas of hypoxia, commonly referred to as "dead zones," where the low level of oxygen in the water makes it impossible for aquatic life to survive. The tainted runoff delivered from the Mississippi to the Gulf of Mexico spurs algal blooms the size of New Jersey, creating the largest dead zone in the world.[11]

For three days in August of 2014, toxic algal blooms in Lake Erie left half a million people in Toledo, Ohio, without a clean drinking water source. The EPA warns of more days with water too dangerous to drink in the years ahead.[12]

Organic certification disallows the use of synthetic fertilizers and chemical pesticides. Organics improve water quality by avoiding unnatural chemicals but certification has no specific requirements regarding water efficiency. A sign posted on a field I often pass reads ORGANIC FARM. DO NOT SPRAY. It's not uncommon to see groundwater, however, being sprayed over these organic fields from tall sprinkler heads, rain or shine. Often the sprinklers are on during the hottest time of day,

---

10. Maude Barlow, *Blue Covenant: The Global Water Crisis and the Coming Battle for the Right to Water* (New York: New Press, 2007).
11. Christine Dell'Amore, "Biggest Dead Zone Ever Forecast in Gulf of Mexico," *National Geographic*, June 24, 2013, http://news.nationalgeographic.com/news/2013/06/130621-dead-zone-biggest-gulf-of-mexico-science-environment.
12. "Status of Nutrients in the Lake Erie Basin," US EPA Lake Erie Nutrient Science Task Group, 2010.

when water loss due to evaporation is at its peak. Sprinklers are second only to flood irrigation as the most inefficient method of irrigation to water crops.

The cabbage found in the organic section of the supermarket might in fact be grown by the same producer as the non-organic variety. I use cabbage as an example because the organic farm I just mentioned grows cabbage, as does the field directly across the road from it, which is marked with a sign that reads DANGER, DO NOT ENTER. This farm had been sprayed with chemicals.

One day I stopped at the organic field and approached a farmworker making her way to her car at the close of the day.

"Do you know who owns the field across the road?" I pointed to the straight lines of conventionally grown cabbage.

"Yes," she said. "It has the same owner as this field."

~

"Better for water" is not enough. I want the best for water. This desire led me to my local farmers' market, a feast for the senses unmatched by the aisles of a supermarket. Orange dahlias were abloom, chunks of goat cheese swam in marinades of oil, and heirloom tomatoes sparkled in the sun, so hearty and ripe they seemed ready to burst from their skins. On one visit I spoke to a woman selling marinated olives flecked with oregano and thyme and almonds bathed in coconut milk.

"Where are your olives and almonds grown?" I asked her.

"In the Central Valley," she replied.

The Central Valley, located in the center of California, is the top producer of fruit, vegetables, and milk in the nation. It also accounts for one-sixth of all irrigated land in the US.[13] The incessant excavation

13. Thomas E. Reilly et al., "Ground-Water Availability in the United States," US Geological Survey, *Circular* 1323: 84.

of water for irrigation left more than 1,000 families in the small agricultural community of East Porterville without running water, when their shallow wells went dry.

"How do you irrigate your trees?"

"We don't. We dry farm."

"My father and brother are the farmers in the family. If you visit the farm, they can show you."

So came the idea to visit farms.

One of my first farm visits following my conversation with the woman at the farmers' market was to John DeRosier's With the Grain farm, in Paso Robles, California. He is a dry farmer growing a diversity of grains without irrigation during the winter and even summer months, when the temperature consistently tops 110 degrees.

He had to explain it to me several times; the concept seemed implausible to me. "How is it you can farm without irrigation while all the neighboring farms are drilling 1,000 feet beneath the surface?" I pointed to the surrounding sea of grapevines clinging to the soft hillsides.

"It starts with the cover crop," he told me. He took me to a field planted with purple flowers. "This is vetch," he told me. "It's a legume like a peanut that transfers nitrogen from the air into the soil." I was amazed that such a beautiful field of wildflowers was busy feeding the soil.

Cover crop is important, I learned from John, because the decaying plant material from the cover crop feeds the bacteria in the soil. This process builds the soil organic matter (SOM). SOM can retain up to 1,000 times more water than soil lacking it, according to the United States Department of Agriculture (USDA) Natural Resources Conservation Services. While his neighbors drill deeper wells to irrigate wine grapes and almond trees, John's crops grow with the moisture held at the surface between the granules of soil. Only 3 percent of American farms reported growing cover crops in the latest Census of Agriculture, and the practice drops with farms larger than 200 acres.

As we walked across the field, John posed me a riddle, "Well-meaning people will order a soy burger instead of a hamburger thinking it's more environmentally friendly as well as a healthier choice. Sometimes it's true, but sometimes it's not. What if the soy used in the veggie burger comes from irrigated fields, but the beef is from rain-fed, pasture-raised cows?"

To answer this riddle for you, first I must introduce the concept of water "color." Water footprint researchers differentiate water sources by assigning them colors: blue, green, and gray. Blue water is sourced from aquifers, reservoirs and all the rivers that scribble across the landscape. Rainwater and fog is green. Gray is water tainted with nitrogen, the runoff from fertilizer and manure.

If we consider water footprint totals alone, then the soy burger, with a water footprint of 224 gallons per pound, is a superior choice. But if the soy burger originates in a field irrigated by ground or surface water, it has a water footprint of 224 gallons of *blue* water, plus unknown gallons of *gray* water if grown on fields treated with chemicals fertilizers. If the pound of hamburger is from a cow fed a diet of rain-fed grass, it's 1,851 gallons of *green* water, rain. Even with an overall higher water footprint total, the rain-fed beef hamburger is better for water preservation in the long run—that is, of course, assuming the pasture is not overgrazed or carved from forests.[14]

Since my farm tour with John, I've interviewed twenty farm owners and ranchers, one chocolatier, a master gardener, a fisherman, a tequila and winemaker, and three brewers. They each taught me ways that food can be grown water-sustainably.

I define "water-sustainable" as food raised or produced using methods that minimally divert the natural progression of water, the supply.

14. See "Chapter 10: Meat & Water" for an in-depth discussion on the best ways to raise animals for water and forests.

In the chapters that follow, you will learn as I did that farm methods focused on developing soil health need little to no irrigation.

Water-sustainable food can even *improve* water quality, as I found at Cobblestone Farm in Upstate New York. Paul and Maureen Knapp converted their dairy to organic after learning the river carved in their land was at the headwaters of the Chesapeake watershed. The Chesepeake is home to the first dead zone discovered in the US, a hypoxic zone that spread over 40 percent of the Chesapeake.[15] At least 50 percent of such pollution stems from agriculture upstream.[16]

Paul and Maureen's concern for water quality led them to implement holistic management, a farm method of corralling animals into small areas of pasture or paddock that are frequently relocated to eliminate overgrazing.

"Before we implemented holistic management, the grass dried out in the summer, and we had to supplement their feed with soybeans. Now the cows rely solely on the pasture," Maureen told me. The soybeans were sourced from irrigated fields treated with glyphosate.

"Why doesn't the grass dry out now?" I asked.

Maureen explained how more vegetative cover and fewer bare spots of land were left behind when the animals are moved off each paddock quicker. The vegetative cover provides the necessary conditions for new seeds to germinate to replenish the grass.

Just like John DeRosier's cover crop, the soil at Cobblestone Farms is rich with organic matter. Both farms retain up to 1,000 times more water than farms that use conventional farming methods.

15. Darryl Fears, "Alarming 'dead zone' grows in the Chesapeake," *Washington Post*, July 24, 2011, https://www.washingtonpost.com/national/health-science/alarming-dead-zone-grows-in-the-chesapeake/2011/07/20/gIQABRmKXI_story.html?utm_term=.3a72b0b4c823.

16. Claudia Copeland, "Animal Waste and Water Quality: EPA's Response to the Waterkeeper Alliance Court Decision on Regulation of CAFOs," Rep. no. 7-5700, Congressional Research Service, 2011.

Crops are thirstier for water when farm acres are treated with chemical fertilizers and pesticides because the poison diminishes the organic matter in the soil. Yet the USDA reports 91 percent of harvested farm acres are sprayed or dusted with herbicides alone.[17] This total does not include private and public lawns and gardens treated with chemicals like Roundup Ready.

"Farmers are water managers. It is my job to keep every drop of water staying where it falls," said Alfred Farris, an organic, no-till farmer in Tennessee, who has experimented with various sustainable farming practices for over forty years. Every person I interviewed for this book is a water manager, each a curator of the land and water.

In the following chapters, I take you with me to these farms, whose products represent the most popular foods and beverages consumed in the United States. I include questions I asked in the hope you'll ask similar questions of your food producers. If more of us ask questions, I have no doubt more food producers will become water managers.

At the end of every chapter, I've included recipes given to me by farmers or food producers showcased in the chapters and some are my own. The recipes are included to give you a starting point to "eat less water."

"You must be the change you want to see in the world," India's Mahatma Gandhi taught. Today, every river in India is polluted, and groundwater levels shrink from over-pumping to grow food for export and to feed India's billions. It's a pattern increasingly common around the world. The crisis is at hand, yet few of us are aware of it or understand how our behavior contributes to it.

---

17. "Table 49. Fertilizers and Chemicals Applies: 2012 and 2007," USDA National Agricultural Statistics Service, 2014, https://www.agcensus.usda.gov/Publications/2012/Full_Report/Volume_1,_Chapter_1_US. According to 2012 figures, 314,964,600 acres were harvested (refer to table 9). I used this figure to calculate the percentage based on the reporting of 285,510,954 "acres treated to control weeds grass or brush" (refer to table 49). Thirty-two percent of harvested cropland is treated with insecticides.

Each of us can be the change we want to see by modifying our wasteful habits; we can preserve and conserve freshwater resources now and for future generations. What we choose to put on our dinner tables can rewrite the story of water scarcity touching people around the world.

Be part of a change that will make a difference in creeks, rivers, groundwater, and oceans across the planet. Start tonight at your kitchen table.

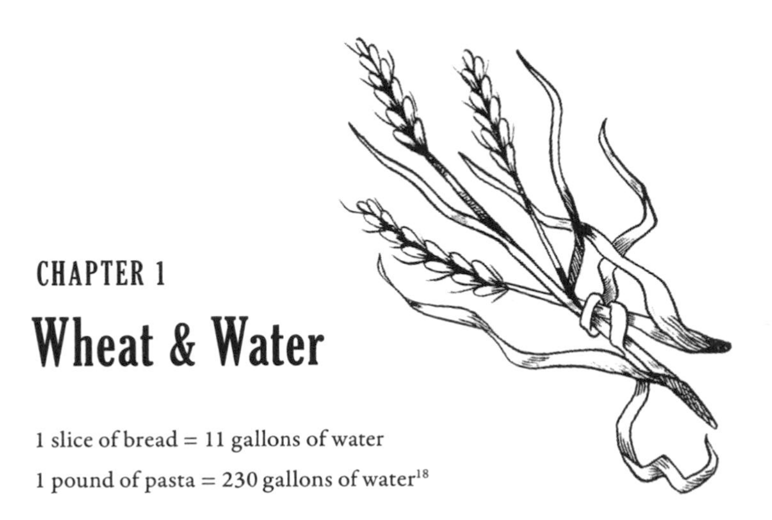

CHAPTER 1

Wheat & Water

1 slice of bread = 11 gallons of water

1 pound of pasta = 230 gallons of water[18]

THE AVERAGE AMERICAN eats nineteen pounds of pasta each year on average, the equivalent of 4,370 gallons of virtual fresh water. At my kitchen table, homemade pasta noodles pirouette around forks. The sound of chewing replaces the usual chatter. In one sitting, my family of five easily slurps 230 gallons of virtual water, the water footprint of a single pound of pasta.

Ten percent of pasta's principle ingredient, wheat, is grown with groundwater, enough water to fill two Nile Rivers annually. The majority of the world's wheat, 66 percent, requires no irrigation. Instead, wheat—grown on more land than any other crop in the world—is rain-fed, cultivated with *green* water. As the global climate changes, the percentage of irrigated wheat fields will change too.

According to the United Nations World Water Report, Earth will warm anywhere between 2–11.5°F within a century. Warmer temperatures will lead to about 8–10 percent more water cycling around our planet from melted glaciers, enough fresh water to fill twenty Nile Rivers. The extra water in the hydrologic cycle causes rivers to swell, widen, and spill ungracefully onto cropland.

---

18. Thomas Kostigen, *The Green Blue Book: The Simple Water-Savings Guide to Everything in Your Life* (Emmaus, PA: Rodale, 2010).

Conversely, warmer temperatures cause longer periods of severe droughts, reducing crop yields by up to one-third and increasing the need for irrigation. If one of the most widely grown crops in the world demands a larger share of surface and groundwater, what will it mean for already stressed water systems?

The uncertainty of our future climate makes farmer John DeRosier's 200 acres of wheat even more significant. John's farm, With the Grain, is dry farmed. Dry farming is similar to rain-fed agriculture: neither uses irrigation, but dry farming involves more than praying for rain. Dry farmers can farm in regions receiving scant amounts of rainfall, like Paso Robles, California, where John's farm is located.

Rain is imminent on the spring day of my visit, but rain is scarce in this region of the world, which receives less rainfall than the desert city of Phoenix, Arizona. Wheat crops need annual rainfall of ten inches or more, or the farmer floods the fields with water, turning fields of wheat into shallow lakes. Flood irrigation equipment is cheaper than sprinklers or drip lines, but the water loss through runoff and evaporation is the highest amongst all forms of irrigation.

"You don't irrigate your crops even in the dry months or during droughts?" I ask John. Dust covers his faded hat and jacket, giving the impression he is older than his years. The brightness in his light blue eyes gives his youth away.

"I don't need to. You can come out onto my field in the summer and see dry, cracked topsoil, but just underneath the soil is moist. My soil retains hundreds of thousands of gallons of water when it rains."

"Why don't you need groundwater to grow your grain?" John has told me his well maintains the same level as when it was drilled six decades earlier: 300 feet. Surrounding vineyards are drilling 1,000 feet beneath the surface to find water. These wells act like big straws, slurping up water from the aquifers for irrigation. When they dry up, deeper wells replace them.[19]

"Your answer starts with cover crop." He leads me down the slope to his "dirt laboratory," slender strips of land used to experiment with new grain varieties.

"This is where the elegance of the farm begins," he smiles. We stand next to a patch of clumpy grass mixed with legumes and peas abloom with periwinkle-blue flowers.

"This is cover crop?" I point down at the grass.

"Yes, grass is the most important thing we got going on, on our planet." He yanks out a chunk of grass, exposing its dangling strings of thin roots.

"Before the rain, I turn the cover crop, incorporating these root systems combined with the tap root of the legumes into the soil. The rainwater infiltrates into the soil and is held in the pores and roots."

"Why don't more farms grow cover crops?" I ask.

"Cover cropping requires more time and double the land. For example, my 200 acres are carved into plots. Half the plots are planted with grain and the other with a cover crop. Each plot is on a two-year cycle alternating between both."

"You produce grain on only half of your acreage at any given time?"

"Correct, but remember I can grow on land other farmers consider unsuitable for farming because there's no water source."

We move to a large field. It looks like a giant plate of chocolate cake. John squats close to the ground and scoops the soil with his hand. It is sprinkled with flecks of ground cover.

"This plot here is breaking down the cover crop. The roots are feeding the microorganisms, bacteria that work to convert nitrogen from the

---

19. In 2014, California passed legislation to regulate groundwater. The law will not be fully enacted until 2040.

air into nitrogen the plant can use. Gazillions of these microorganisms lie underground in the humus."

Humus is another name for soil with organic matter (SOM). It retains more moisture than synthetic or even organic soils. A report published by *Soil Science* found humus to hold water at 80–90 percent of its weight.[20]

Humus isn't present on all farms. When soil is chemically treated the microorganisms are eradicated along with weeds and pests. The living organisms in humus, like the crops, need to be cultivated with patience and planning.

"You never add fertilizers?" I ask. In my backyard garden, I'm accustomed to mixing bags of fertilizer in my soil before every new planting.

"No. I don't import fertilizer. It is the biggest distinction between the organic and the biodynamic farmer."

The word "biodynamic" is new to me.

"A biodynamic farmer sees the farm as a living system that works in coordination, like the organs of the body." Biodynamic farming recognizes the natural pattern and rhythm of nature. Developed by Rudolf Steiner in 1924, it's similar to organic farming. Chemicals, synthetic fertilizers and GMO seeds are disallowed, but in addition to organic standards, biodynamics encompasses a framework designed to build biological diversity. When everything comes together, the farm is self-sufficient, requiring little to no external farm *inputs* such as fertilizers, seeds, and water.

"This farm produces its fertilizer through cover crop, crop rotation, and manure from the animals raised on the farm," John adds. "If you import nutrients with the purchase of fertilizers, you're not bound by crop rotation."

---

20. Alan Olness and David Archer, "Effect of organic carbon on available water in soil," *Soil Science* 170 (2005): 90–101.

The first raindrops begin to fall. John has been up since 4:00 a.m. preparing his land to receive the rain.

"To farm this way, my timing needs to be impeccable. If rain is on the way, I need to be ready to turn the soil, no matter what time of day or night it is."

"So this is rugged farming?" I ask.

He laughs. "Yes, this is on-the-edge farming." He pauses. "But I wouldn't do it any other way."

Joaquin's Favorite Homemade Pasta

Makes 8 servings

40 minutes to prepare

3 minutes to cook

Our Italian machine grows long linguine noodles with ease. My three young children wait their turn to crank the dough through the pasta machine. Each noodle is dusted with gold, coarse semolina flour. Fresh pasta falls limply into boiling salted water. Out of the pot, I dress the naked linguine with sautéed tomatoes, garlic, basil, and shreds of parmesan married with two ladlefuls of pasta water. I can count on my son Joaquin staying at the table long after we've all left, slurping noodles until they're gone.

The key to water-sustainable pasta is the choice of flour. If you buy from a local farm, ask if the wheat is irrigated. If the answer is yes, the follow-up question is how often and with what irrigation method (remember, flood irrigation is the least efficient). If you purchase flour from a grocer, notice the region where it's grown. For example, North Dakota, South Dakota, and Montana are rain-fed regions.

This recipe can be used with or without a pasta machine. The pasta machine I use is the Marcato Atlas 150.

Ingredients

2 cups dry-farmed or rain-fed organic flour

2 cups dry-farmed or rain-fed organic semolina flour

1 pinch salt
6 large farm-fresh rotationally pastured organic eggs[21]
2 tablespoons organic olive oil (look for dry farmed)

Directions

1. Sift together the flour, semolina flour, and salt into a medium bowl and combine.
2. Make a deep well in the center of the dry ingredients.
3. In a separate bowl, whisk the eggs and oil.
4. Pour the mixture into the center and, with your hands, fold the dry and wet ingredients together.
5. Once folded, pour onto a surface dusted with flour. Knead the dough until it is smooth and supple, about 8–10 minutes.
6. Wrap the dough tightly in plastic wrap and leave it at room temperature for 30 minutes.
7. Roll the dough to your desired thickness and cut it into your favorite noodle shape, or refer to the directions provided with your pasta machine.
8. Place the fresh pasta on a counter dusted with semolina or hang it on plastic hangers to keep noodles from sticking to each other.
9. Boil enough water to cover the noodles, 2 quarts for a pound of pasta (trust me, this is all the water you need, not the 4–6 quarts suggested.) Add 1 tablespoon of salt for every quart of water to season the pasta. Add pasta noodles into the boiling water, making sure they are separate pieces, not one big clump. Stir a few times to be sure the pasta does not stick together. Fresh pasta cooks fast, so stay close. Check to see if it's done at 3 minutes, if it's not done, keep checking at 1-minute intervals.
10. Remove the pasta from the water. Save the pasta water to make your favorite sauce. Reusing pasta water in sauces is common

---

21. See "Chapter 7: Eggs & Water."

practice in Italy. The starchy, salty water is excellent in pasta sauces; it thins the sauce and adds a rich, buttery flavor. You'll find yourself wiping the plate clean.

Mama's Whole Wheat Bread

Makes 3 loaves

45 minutes to prepare plus rise time

30 minutes to bake

Most weeks, I bake our family bread. The kids call it Mama's Bread. The steam rises from the slices of fresh-baked bread when lathered with generous amounts of butter and drizzles of honey. I can count on one loaf disappearing the first day. The second loaf is reserved for the week's sandwiches. The third loaf is frozen for the following week's sandwiches.

I control the source of the ingredients when I bake my bread. The flour is organic and originates from North Dakota and Montana, two states exclusively rain-fed (I emailed the manufacturers to confirm this information). The butter is made from milk from pasture-raised cows (see "Chapter 9: Dairy & Water"). Our honey is from a neighbor who ladles the golden delight straight from the hive.

Ingredients

- 3 cups warm water
- 2 (0.25 ounce) packages active dry yeast
- ⅔ cup organic local honey
- 5 cups unbleached organic dry-farmed or rain-fed white flour
- 3½ cups organic dry-farmed or rain-fed wheat flour
- 3 tablespoons organic pastured butter, melted
- 1 tablespoon salt

2 additional tablespoons organic butter melted reserved for the bread out of the oven

Directions

1. Preheat oven to 375°F.
2. Mix warm water, yeast and ⅓ cup honey (reserve the additional ⅓ cup honey for later in the recipe) and 5 cups white organic flour. Stir ingredients to combine.
3. Set the bowl aside for 30 minutes or until bubbles appear.
4. Mix in 3 tablespoons melted butter, the remaining ⅓ cup honey and salt.
5. Stir in 2 cups of the wheat flour to begin. Flour a clean surface with whole wheat flour and knead. Add an additional 2–4 cups whole wheat flour one cup at a time. Knead the dough until it's no longer sticky.
6. Place the round, smooth dough into a greased bowl to keep it from sticking. Cover with a dishtowel to keep out drafts. Leave the dough to rise. The dough will double in size.
7. Punch the dough after it has risen (I love this part). Divide the dough into equal parts.
8. Grease three 9×5-inch loaf pans. I use butter to grease, but you can use oil too. Place the dough in the pans and allow the dough to rise a second time. You know the dough is ready when it rises above the tops of the pans. If you don't have loaf pans, hand-form the dough. Stretch the dough out to resemble the shape of a loaf of bread and place on a greased cookie sheet.
9. Bake for 25–30 minutes or until the bread has a hollow sound when tapped with a wooden spoon. Lightly brush the tops of the loaves with 2 tablespoons melted butter to prevent the crust from hardening.

CHAPTER 2

Rice & Water

1 cup of cooked rice = 50 gallons of water

1 pound of uncooked rice = 300 gallons of water[22]

RICE, THE MOST consumed staple on earth, provides one-fifth of the world's caloric intake. It is spiced with saffron, sprinkled with soy sauce, paired with red beans. To feed a growing population, yields must double by 2050 to feed 2.4 billion more people.[23] Rice currently consumes 30 percent of all surface and drinking water.[24] It will require twice the water to grow double the rice. Where will the water come from?

Two sizable barriers stand in the way of bigger yields: climate change and water scarcity. The International Water Management Institute estimates with each 1°C (1.8°F) temperature increase, yields decline by 7 percent. The warmer temperatures impact the availability of water for food crops. Over the next few decades, experts predict water shortages for 25 percent of *irrigated* rice fields. These rice paddies are responsible for growing three-quarters of the world's rice.

---

22. A.K. Chapagain and A.Y. Hoekstra, "The blue, green and grey water footprint of rice from production and consumption perspectives," *Ecological Economics* 70 (2011): 749–58. You can download this study and others at http://www.waterfootprint.org.
23. "World population projected to reach 9.6 billion by 2050—UN report," *UN News Centre*, June 13, 2013, http://www.un.org/apps/news/story.asp?NewsID=45165#.WGwWu9IrIY1. The world population in 2013 was 7.2 billion. The United Nations projects the total to increase to 9.6 billion by 2050, with the majority of the population growth occurring in the forty-nine least developed nations.
24. Chapagain and Hoekstra, "The blue, green and grey water footprint of rice."

Globally, ten million small family farms grow rice with 40 percent less water than the average flooded rice field. Their rice cultivation method, known as the System of Rice Intensification (SRI), produces stronger plants which are more resistant to extreme weather and have lower arsenic and methane levels endemic to flooded rice.[25]

The United States is home to only three farms implementing SRI.[26] A staff member of SRI International Network and Resource Center located at Cornell University helped me find one of them, three hours from New Orleans.

Kurt Unkel, the owner of Cajun Grain Rice, dashes around his warehouse in the small downtown of Kinder, Louisiana. He pieces together his stone mill used to grind rice into grits or cracked rice. His son Seth works in the far corner of the lofty room repairing another stone mill, paying little attention to his father's constant motion.[27] With all the pieces gathered, Kurt scoops the rice into the shelling machine to remove the hull, the protective hard case embracing each grain. The rice falls into the machine, the sound like a rain stick. Next, he grinds the brown jasmine rice stripped of the hull, but complete with its layer of bran. Kurt holds the ground rice out for me to inhale.

"It's awesome that first smell," says Kurt. The scent is hard to describe, except with words like "soft" and "cozy."

"What does it smell like to you?" I ask Kurt.

"It smells like rice to me. I've been in this for all my life." His shoulders on his lanky frame rise and fall with the rhythm of his laughter.

Kurt digs deep without any prompting. "When I started farming, I couldn't grow anything without fertilizers," he tells me while reaching

25. "More Rice for People, More Water for the Planet: System of Rice Intensification (SRI)," Africare, Oxfam America, WWF-ICRISAT Project (2010), Online at http://www.sri-india.net/documents/More_Water_For_The_Planet.pdf

26. Chapagain and Hoekstra, "The blue, green and grey water footprint of rice." The United States ranks eleventh in top-producing rice countries. China, India and Indonesia are the world's top producers.

27. Kurt Unkel and Seth Unkel in discussion with the author, August 2014.

for the Cajun Grain labels to glue on the bags of fresh rice flour and grits he's grounded for me.

"There was no fertility left in the soil. We've grown rice here for 100 years, but we can't grow rice on the land no more without adding fertilizers. We've depleted the land. But nature can put the fertility all back. The good Lord made all this work. Now I can grow anything."

I follow him into his office space adjoining the nearly completed industrial kitchen where he plans to host cooking classes and prepare healthy, flavorful pre-packaged meals for local pick-up.

"When you start to grow a plant, 95 percent of its growth is going to come from the air and about 5 percent from the soil. So why dump millions of pounds of fertilizers on the land? The plant is carbon, nitrogen, and oxygen. Where does that come from? It comes out of the air. It's all free." Kurt outstretches his arms into the open air and smiles.

Ninety-five percent of the plant's dry weight is carbon, hydrogen, and oxygen. Plants draw in these compounds from the soil through tousled root hairs, but the majority is absorbed through its leaves.[28]

"You start getting the ratios right in the soil—the calcium ratios, phosphorus ratios—then the plant gets it right. When you eat it, *you* get it right. For us to be healthy, the plants need to be healthy."

28. Ray V. Herren, *The Science of Agriculture: A Biological Approach* (Albany, NY: Delmar Thomson Learning, 1997). In the 1600s, Dutchman Jan Baptista van Helmont set out to learn how a tree derived its weight. He observed the growth of a willow tree in a container for five years. In the beginning of the experiment the willow tree weighed 5 pounds and the soil 200 pounds. No inputs of fertilizer or water were added. The tree, placed outside, was watered with natural rain. At the conclusion of the experiment the willow gained 160 pounds and the soil lost 2 ounces. He concluded the weight of the tree was from the water and explained the 2 ounce loss of soil to an error in soil weight at the inception of the experiment. With subsequent research, he found that although he was right to conclude the weight of the tree was not from the soil, it did not arise from the water. Most of the weight is due to the absorption of carbon dioxide. The soil did in fact lose 2 ounces of weight. The change of weight is explained by the tree's absorption of minerals in the soil. The most essential nutrients, referred to as macronutrients, are in mineral and non-mineral form. They include the non-minerals of carbon, oxygen, hydrogen and the minerals of nitrogen, phosphorus, potassium, sulfur, calcium, and magnesium.

According to the USDA nutritional composition tables, fruits and vegetables have fewer vitamins and minerals than they did in 1975. Broccoli has lost 54 percent of its calcium, iron levels are down 60 percent in cauliflower and apples, and bananas have 48 percent less phosphorus on average.[29]

"How do you know if the ratios are right in the soil?"

"You test the nutrients available to the plant with a soil test."

I follow him to his desk. He pulls the test results from a stack of papers on his desktop and places his reading glasses on the edge of his nose. He holds the paper where both of us can examine it.

"This shows me what's in the soil. For example, this here is the calcium results." He points to the first column of numbers. "The soil had 2,000 parts per million of calcium, but what's available to the plant is only 500 parts per million. So my question is why is the calcium tied up and what do I need to do differently to make the nutrient available to the plant?"

Soil tests are encouraged for farmers and home gardeners alike to foster healthy plant growth and reduce nutrient runoff, the largest source of pollution of US waterways. For a minimal fee, soil tests measure the elements available to the plant. Based on the soil sample, recommendations of phosphorus, potassium, and nitrogen are tailored to address nutrient deficiencies.

"Keep putting only nitrogen, phosphorus, and potassium on the ground year after year, and it throws your ratios out off balance. When your ratios get out of balance, you get more weeds. You get more weeds, you got to put on more chemicals to kill them, but the chemicals kill the

29. There are exceptions to the decline (carrots and pumpkins) but overall declines are reported in vitamins and minerals for nearly every fruit and vegetable. I compared 2015 totals to 1975. You can find updated USDA results with the following link to the National Nutrient Database for Standard Reference: http://ndb.nal.usda.gov/ndb. A partial list of USDA fruit and vegetables nutrition level results from 1975 are found in the following report also available online: Alex Jack, "America's Vanishing Nutrients: Decline in Fruit and Vegetable Quality Poses Serious Health and Environmental Risks," (2005), http://rockdustlocal.com/uploads/3/4/3/4/34349856/americas_vanishing_nutrients.pdf.

bacteria. It's a chain reaction." Kurt puts the soil test results down, takes off his reading glasses, and adjusts his faded baseball cap.

The end goal of repeated soil testing in a ratio system is for the plant to thrive without fertilizers. Like the standard soil test, the ratios test measures the amount of nutrients available to the plant, but it also measures the nutrients present in the soil. Based on the results, a recommendation of *inputs* is given to the farmer/gardener. The standard recommendations of nitrogen, phosphorus, and potassium, (NPK) are passed over for inputs that cultivate bacteria and fungi in soil like lime, fish fertilizer, and molasses. Bacteria and fungi naturally bring minerals to the plant by breaking down and dispersing decomposed plant material.[30] NPK found in all commercial fertilizer mixes leave salt deposits that kill the fungi and bacteria in soil, requiring the reapplication of fertilizers with every planting.

"I think there are five major fertilizer companies worldwide. They pump millions of dollars to develop this stuff. They don't want to develop anything that's not going to make them no money. And it costs us. We lost our soil, and we lost our health."

The top five chemical fertilizer companies, each with facilities in the US, account for 33 percent of the world market share. PotashCorp, the largest among them, grosses more than a billion dollars annually.[31]

~

Kurt, his son Seth, and I climb into his Trailblazer to grab "dinner" (Southern for lunch) before the farm visit. They choose Fausto's Fam-

30. Joe Miazgowicz (Crop Services International) in discussion with the author, January 2015.

31. "Q3: PotashCorp Reports Third-Quarter Earnings of $0.38 per Share," PotashCorp: Helping Nature Provide, October 23, 2014, http://www.potashcorp.com/news/1916. The 33 percent figure is according to data released by a marketing research firm for 2012. The full report can be found at http://www.lucintel.com/reports/chemical_composites/top_five_global_fertilizer_companies_performance_strategies_and_competitive_analysis.aspx.

ily Restaurant because I'd asked for local cuisine. A twelve-foot stuffed alligator is prominently displayed on the far wall. It blends into the furniture for most patrons, except for a few small children and me, the only tourist, who can't resist gawking.

Crawfish is a popular item among the extensive meal choices posted on the wall.

"Do you grow crawfish?" I ask Kurt while we wait our turn. Production of the tasty crustaceans stretches over 180,000 acres of land in Louisiana.[32] Many rice farmers down here harvest crawfish on their flooded fields. The income generated by the small freshwater crustaceans keep smaller rice farmers afloat.[33]

"I think the crawfish pull too much out of the soil. Crawfish eat the microbes in the soil. Since I'm rebuilding my soil, I don't want to take anything away. When you take the crawfish off your land, you pull minerals and microbes out with them. To be a true organic, sustainable farmer you need to give more than you take." He pauses between the final five words.

The ebb and flow of water on rice fields is a natural breeding ground for crawfish. They grow in shallow fresh water and burrow into the mud when the field is drawn down or *dewatered*. Crawfish ponds are flooded nine times per season to maintain good water quality, six to seven more times than a typical rice field. The increased flooding puts additional demands on water supplies, principally groundwater.[34]

---

32. Dr. Ray McClain (Louisiana State University Rice Research Station) in discussion with the author, December 2014.

33. Dave Thier, "In Louisiana, Growing Rice to Trade on Some Creatures That Eat It," *New York Times*, December 5, 2012, http://www.nytimes.com/2012/12/06/us/in-louisiana-farmers-use-rice-fields-as-crayfish-ponds.html?_r=0.

34. W. Ray McClain et al., "Louisiana Crawfish Production Manual," no. 2637, LSU AgCenter, January 2007, http://www.lsuagcenter.com/NR/rdonlyres/3AD14F0D-567D-4334-B572-D55D1C55A1F1/34429/pub2637CrawfishProductionManualLOWRES.pdf. Charles Lutz et al., "Crawfish Environmental Best Management Practices," no. 3186, July 2011: 1–28, http://www.lsuagcenter.com/portals/communications/publications/publications_catalog/environment/best%20management%20practices/crawfish-environmental-best-management-practices.

We take our seats in the back dining room under the watchful eyes of elk, wild boar, and buffalo mounted along every wall. "Where does the water come from in this region?" I ask.

Seth answers, "We got a lot of rivers here, and there's a canal system. Drain ditches during my grandpa's day were fifty feet wide and had time to build the water table. The drain ditches would overflow and return nutrients into the soil. Now the drain ditches are thirty feet deep and six feet wide. It's about getting the water out of the way as fast as possible to keep areas from flooding. But everything goes with it—topsoil, pollution and nutrients—and dumps into the Mississippi." Seth pauses as the waitress delivers his baked potato overflowing with shrimp from the Gulf of Mexico. "Now we got a dead zone off our coast from the nutrient runoff from the Mississippi."

The dead zone in the Gulf of Mexico, the largest in the world, grows with continuous deliveries of nutrient-rich water from the Mississippi River. Like the canal system Seth describes during his grandpa's day, the floodwaters of the Mississippi used to carry nutrients like nitrogen and phosphorus to the soil. Today the Mississippi is the most controlled river in the world. Once characterized by Mark Twain as a "lawless stream," it now follows a restricted route defined by 3,600 levees.[35] Its nutrient-rich water swept out to sea.

"Do farmers use the water from the canal system to flood their fields?" I ask. Surface water is a renewable resource, versus groundwater that's experiencing a nationwide drop in levels.

"Everybody got well water around here," says Kurt, as he scoops a forkful of potato from the skin.

---

35. The full Mark Twain quote from *Life on the Mississippi* is the following: "One who knows the Mississippi will promptly aver—not aloud, but to himself—that ten thousand River Commissions, with the mines of the world at their back, cannot tame that lawless stream, cannot curb it or confine it, cannot say to it, Go here, or Go there, and make it obey; cannot save a shore which it has sentenced; cannot bar its path with an obstruction which it will not tear down, dance over, and laugh at."

Kurt explains why farmers favor groundwater over surface water. "It all comes down to economics," he says. Louisiana farmers pay a percentage of their yield, at a rate of about 15–20 percent, to a water company in exchange for unlimited surface water delivery. Farmers, squeezed by increasing costs of fertilizers and seeds, can reduce their costs by eliminating the need for surface water delivery. An estimated 54 percent of water used to irrigate crops is pumped from the ground, while 5 percent is surface water.[36]

~

"Why is arsenic an issue for rice farms?" I ask on the drive to Kurt's farm. Rice accumulates arsenic in the bran layer of the grain.

"In college during the '70s, they'd tell us don't worry about what you put on the land. As long as it's a low enough dose, it won't hurt anything. That's what most people did. They used arsenic for parasite and insect control for cotton and everything else you could grow."

Arsenic, a semi-metallic element, is part of the Earth's crust. First released into the air through a variety of human operations including pesticide spraying, wood preservation, smelting of heavy metals, and coal burning, it eventually settles into the soil and water. In the atmosphere, arsenic is toxic to humans and a known carcinogen.

"It was legal for the fertilizer companies to sell arsenic to farmers. You do that for forty years, and these heavy metals build up and you never get rid of them. The big chemical companies still dump poison on developing nations where they don't have any regulations," Kurt says.

---

36. "Managing Louisiana's Groundwater Resources: With Supplemental Information on Surface Water Resources," Louisiana Ground Water Resources Commission, March 15, 2012, http://dnr.louisiana.gov/assets/docs/conservation/groundwater/12.Final.GW.Report.pdf. In Louisiana, agriculture and aquaculture combined account for 54 percent of aquifer water draws.

Long-term exposure to arsenic causes several cancers, cardiovascular diseases, and diabetes according to the World Health Organization (WHO). *Inorganic* arsenic, a toxic compound, was banned in the US in 1988 after a century of use. The *organic* arsenic compound deemed *less harmful* by the FDA remains legal. *Organic* arsenic is currently applied on golf courses, sod farms, and highway medians. As recent as 2015, the arsenic drug nitarsone was fed to US poultry to prevent parasitic diseases, to encourage faster weight gain, and to give the meat a "healthy" pink coloring.[37] While the *organic* arsenic compound is regarded as nontoxic at the time of application, in aquatic sediment, like flooded rice fields, it converts back into the toxic *inorganic* form.[38]

"A lot of people are blaming flood irrigation for the high levels of heavy metals. If that's the case, then if you can grow the rice with less water, you can lower the risks from heavy metals."

Studies support Kurt's intuition. Rice grown on non-flooded paddies accumulates lower amounts of arsenic and other heavy metals. His own fields, tested by Dillard University, tested well below the Louisiana State limit of 12 mg/kg of arsenic.

~

The loud hum of cicadas is broken by the crunch of gravel underfoot as we hike out to the rice paddies. Seth tells me to stop. "These plots were planted at the same time. You see how the plants on the right side are way taller than the left?"

I nod.

---

37. In recent years, drug manufacturers removed three arsenic drugs used for decades in poultry feed from the US market. The drugs remain available to poultry farmers in Latin America.

38. "Biomonitoring Summary: Arsenic," National Biomonitoring Program, http://www.cdc.gov/biomonitoring/Arsenic_BiomonitoringSummary.html.

"Seth continues the left side was the broadcast part, the seeds thrown out by hand to sprout on the field. Broadcasting the seed is how everyone does it around here. The SRI plot on the right sprouted in containers. We let the seeds grow for five or six days then plant sprout by hand." The color of stalks on the SRI plot are a deeper green and a foot taller than the plot with broadcasted seed.

"Why does planting the sprouted seed versus broadcasting seeds save water?"

"When they're broadcast you end up with ten seeds per square foot on average. By hand I plant only one seed per square foot. So it takes less seed and less water. I may spend $100 an acre hand planting, but I'm going to save $200 an acre on chemicals and fertilizers," Seth tells me.

"It's the importance of first life," Kurt adds. "In those first ten days you make an environment where the plant has all its nutritional needs met and, therefore, grows bigger and faster. And because of that the grain gets a little bit bigger and fatter. When you add a micro ounce to each grain, it adds up," we move along the path, passing the home he shares with his wife Karen.

"Cornell University has studied the SRI rice. They've seen a 50 percent increase in yields under this type of program. With that increase, you can cut your rice crop in half, plant half the land, use half as much of everything, and make more food," Kurt says.

"And use half the water," I add. The connections between this method and water conservation come into focus.

"Even though rice can grow submerged underwater, it does better if oxygen reaches its roots. With SRI rice you let the soil dry up and crack, so the roots get oxygen," says Kurt.

"You only flood once with the SRI method?"

"Yes, we flood the field in the beginning and plant the seedling in the mud. We make a trench with a finger and lay the sprout down in the mud and cover the root. The roots will grow down, and the plant will stand," says Kurt.

"As opposed to keeping the field flooded for long periods of time as is the conventional practice," interjects Seth. "With the SRI method we let the field dry out for short periods and flood for the rest of the life of the rice."

"Do the root systems grow deeper on a non-flooded field?"

The cicadas' hum becomes a roar. Father and son continue, uninterrupted by the summer song.

"With the SRI method, you're giving the soil a chance to rebuild because you're giving the soil oxygen. As you build the soil, the oxygen is available to the roots and the roots can grow deeper. As the root systems grow deeper it makes more root holes, which means more oxygen. Everything feeds off everything," says Kurt.

Seth points to the SRI test plot. "If you pull one of those plants, the root will have a larger ball of roots than with the broadcast rice. The root ball has the same surface area as the part of the plant above the ground. When you have a taller plant, you have a bigger root system."

"Why are rice fields flooded?" I've yet to ask the most obvious question in my search to understand how to save water at the farm.

"Rice needs a tremendous amount of water when it's growing," answers Kurt. "The water level drops an inch a day. But the main purpose for flooding is weed control."

On the walk back to the car, Kurt stops and squats down close to the ground. He digs up soil underneath the compost of decaying grass. He cradles the clumps of dirt in his outstretched hand. "The amount of bacteria in healthy soil is unbelievable. The bacteria make all those little clumps. All them little clumps keep everything from leeching out. Bacteria are 80 percent water. When it rains, the bacteria absorb the water. And as the bacteria naturally die, the water is released. If you want to conserve water, you got to put the life back into the soil. Bacteria will manage the moisture for you." He stands and shakes the dirt from his hand and walks toward the Trailblazer.

Kurt continues, "The bacteria in healthy soil let oxygen in. When the ground gets packed, the air can't get in. Low oxygen is the number one problem with the soil. Think about your own survival. What's the first thing that's going to kill you? No oxygen. Next, what's going to kill you? No water. Next is food. The fertilizer should be the last thing we worry about, but for most farmers it's the first. When you start doing this stuff, you learn the life in the soil needs the same thing we do." His voice lowers to a whisper, "It is a fascinating world." He opens the passenger door, and I slip inside.

We drive a short distance to the 2,500 acres of rice jointly farmed by Kurt's three brothers and nephew. Today is harvest day.

"Does everyone else in your family grow rice conventionally?" I wonder aloud.

"Yes, but one of my brothers tested my fertilizer program on 100 acres. He didn't go organic, he just used fish fertilizer. But he grew rice just as good and cheaper."

"What about your other brothers?"

"My brothers are getting older. The last thing they want to do is start a new learning curve. They're trying to figure what they can do to retire in five to ten years. They don't want to try to introduce a new operation. I think that's the issue for farmers in general."

At the farm, the cherry-red combine harvester is at a standstill awaiting a truck to transfer the overflowing rice. Cattle egrets stand regally behind the combine. Their striking white feathers are framed by the golden hue of the grass.

We get out of the Trailblazer and move into the rice field. The birds take flight.

"Do you want to ride in the combine?" Kurt asks me. I jump at the offer. We get back into the Trailblazer and drive closer to the massive machine.

The combine is loud. The engine swallows half our words. Kurt helps me to the ladder to reach the glass-enclosed cab. Inside is quiet. Kurt leaves me with his young nephew, Aaron, who is in the driver's seat.

The combine begins to roll. The egrets descend toward us, their wings unfurl over the air current and disappear to the rear.

"The cattle egrets catch the grasshoppers when they leap out of the field ahead of the combine," Aaron says.

In one quick motion, the plants are yanked from the ground with the steel teeth and moved up the conveyor. Inside the belly of the machine, the grain is threshed and winnowed; the rice husks litter the ground behind the combine, while the grain falls clean into the tank.

"How much do these machines cost?"

"New, about $400,000. My uncles and I share the cost of the equipment."

"Do you find it's getting more expensive to grow rice?

"The cost of everything is going up. Equipment, everything."

"What do you think about the way your Uncle Kurt is farming?"

"He's doing good." Aaron smiles.

"Have you considered farming like him?

"Naw, I keep doing it the conventional way."

Aaron pulls the combine harvester up beside the Trailblazer. He helps me down, climbs back into the driver's seat and pulls ahead. The egrets follow close behind him.

"I asked your nephew if he has any plans to farm like you," I tell Kurt when we're back in the Trailblazer.

"What did he say?" Kurt's interest piqued.

Kurt shows no surprise when I tell him, but I sense his longing to have his family reconsider the way they farm.

"Something's got to show them there's more money to be made without dependence on government subsidies. Years back, my uncle put a computer program together for me to monitor my expenses. The program showed me how my expenses kept going up every year, farming the conventional way. But the subsidy stayed the same. I saw even then there ain't going to be no future in the old ways."

Seth agrees. "Farmers make the same amount of money they did twenty-five years ago under government subsidy programs. They change the names of the programs with every farm bill, but the money don't change."

Farm subsidies are rooted in the Great Depression administrations of Franklin D. Roosevelt and Herbert Hoover. Farm support of specific commodities, like rice, has become a permanent fixture in US farm bills, though a diverse collection of groups, from economists to environmentalists, has called for their elimination.

In the 2014 Farm Bill, direct payments to farmers were repealed but a heavily subsidized crop insurance-based system replaced them.[39] Long after the Great Depression, American farming is still shaped by government subsidies. The relationship between the farmer and the subsidy mirrors that of the plant and fertilizers: they are both dependent on *external inputs* for survival.

"It takes time to rebuild the soil. And who's going to pay for that transition time?" Kurt asks me. "Farmers are getting older, and their kids don't want to farm. The kids inherit the land and rent it out to farmers without land of their own. As landowners they don't want to pay to build the soil, they figure that's the farmer's responsibility. But the tenant farmer doesn't build fertility, because the land is not his, and

---

39. Laura Collins, "The 2014 Farm Bill Subsidy Reforms Don't Go Far Enough," American Action Forum, February 7, 2014, https://www.americanactionforum.org/research/the-2014-farm-bill-subsidy-reforms-dont-go-far-enough.

all the minerals he gives back to the land he can't take with him. He needs to make a living and can't wait for the soil to rebuild."

I follow Kurt's gaze to the muddy rice fields, reaching for the horizon in every direction.

"Now there's nothing left in the soil. But soil without minerals and nutrients has cost us our health, it cost us our land and I don't know what it's going to take to change," Kurt says in a quiet voice.

"The world is changing," Kurt becomes excited again. "I get visits on my farm from young kids in their twenties. Some want to farm, others just want to learn how to grow their own food and eat healthy. This next generation knows they have a purpose in life. They don't know what it is, but they're going to find it."

His words hang ripe with optimism on the humid air.

Cajun Grain's Brown Rice Pancakes

Makes 8 medium pancakes

5 minutes to prepare

3 minutes to cook

Rice flour can be substituted for corn meal or wheat flours in your favorite recipes. I order my brown rice from Kurt, ten pounds at a time, or purchase SRI-grown rice from brands like Lotus Foods found at most grocery store chains. SRI rice is low in heavy metal levels, conserves water, and is higher in mineral content.

Cajun Grain may be the only rice in the nation with its own playlist. Kurt's wife, Karen, plays music for the rice plants, a list that includes the Beatles' "Here Comes the Sun" and Carole King's hit, "I Feel the Earth Move." Karen is convinced the music helps the rice grow. And although not scientifically proven, I think Cajun Grain's Brown Rice Pancakes are tastier with music on too.

Ingredients

1½ cups SRI rice flour (look for brands like Cajun Grain or Lotus Foods)

1 cup organic milk

1 egg

¼ teaspoon of baking powder

¼ teaspoon of baking soda

¼ teaspoon cinnamon

1 tablespoon organic fair-trade sugar

Optional: Fresh or frozen blueberries, chopped walnuts

Directions

1. Mix all the ingredients in the same bowl until no lumps remain.
2. Oil a pan or griddle and set on medium heat.
3. Pour ¼ cup of batter into the hot pan (when the pan sizzles a drop of water, it is ready). Cook first side for 2 minutes (use timer). Flip and cook the second side for an additional 1 minute.
4. Top with a slice of organic butter, fruit, walnuts and drizzle with organic pure maple syrup.

CHAPTER 3

Produce & Water

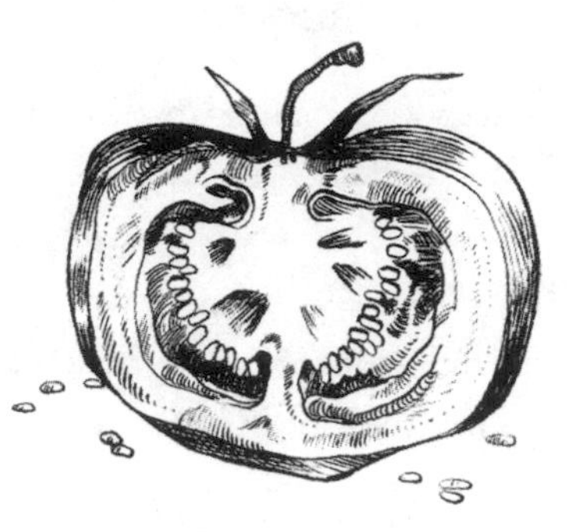

1 pound of lettuce = 10 gallons of water

1 tomato = 13 gallons of water

1 orange = 21 gallons of water

1 apple = 33 gallons of water[40]

A THIN STRIP of rain clouds cuts across the Cascade Mountain range horizontally like a white ribbon. Glacial melt from the mountains washes over the valley floor. The melted snow brings sand, decomposed salmon, and the finest silt to this alluvial flood plain. For this reason, the Skagit Valley is rated among the top 2 percent of the best soils in the world for agricultural production.

But the soil in this "agricultural paradise" is under constant attack from a perpetual mist of chemicals and a global shift in the water cycle.

Nelida Martinez and her grown son, Danny, sow seeds in a hoop house. It is quiet except for the faint sound of ranchera, Mexican folk music, playing at low volume on their battery-operated radio.[41] I unwind my knit scarf inside the warm shelter constructed of wood and plastic.

40. M. M. Mekonnen and A. Y. Hoekstra, "The green, blue and grey water footprint of crops and derived crop products," *Hydrology and Earth System Sciences* 15 (2011): 1577–1600.

41. Nelida Martinez in discussion with the author, March 2014. A special thanks to Leigh Newman-Bell who was present at the interview for as-needed Spanish translation.

"What are you planting?" Nelida and I walk deeper inside the structure. Long, wide tables hold sprouts of vegetables and berries.

"A little of everything." Laughter slips from her easily. She points and names the wide diversity of plants. Strawberry plants resemble three-leaf clovers with fuzzy shoots. Lanky chile sprouts join leafy tomato starts. The bright red stems of chard unfurl green leaves.

Nelida worked as a farmworker before starting her farm, Pura Nelida, meaning "Pure Nelida" in her native Spanish.

She is an unlikely farm owner, but the unlikeliness doesn't stem from inexperience. As a farmworker for twenty years, she learned the different aspects of growing and harvesting food. It is instead her background as a Latina farmworker that makes her leap from worker to owner all the more improbable. In the Skagit Valley, the average farmworker family of four earns $15,229 annually, lower than the federal poverty threshold.[42] The cost to start a farm in Washington State is $30,000.

Nelida Martinez's five acres are leased from Viva Farms, a farm incubator that offers farm equipment and one to five acre parcels at low lease rates after the completion of a three-month course covering all aspects of organic farming.

"Have you always grown organically?" I ask her.

"I've grown food without chemicals since the start. After years in the fields, I know firsthand how chemicals cause physical reactions to the skin and eyes." She pauses. Her words are deliberate. "I imagine those chemicals being absorbed into the body whenever people eat treated vegetables and fruit."

---

42. "Skagit County Farmworker Housing Action Plan: 2010–2015," Washington Farmworker Housing Trust, March 2011. http://web.archive.org/web/20160309064849/http://www.orfh.org/downloads/SkagitActionPlan.pdf. The federal poverty threshold in 2011 was $44,350, the year of the study cited. The federal poverty level in 2017 for a family of four is $30,380.

With 2.5 billion pounds of pesticides used annually in the United States, it is impossible to avoid exposure.[43] We breathe, drink, eat, and roll in grass treated with them. Each of our bodies holds at least 700 chemical contaminants, according to EPA estimates.[44] Farmworkers and growers on the nation's 1.3 million farms have the most intimate and chronic exposure.[45]

"What kind of physical reactions did you experience?"

"I worked on big farms that used a lot of chemicals. The managers got us on the land as soon as possible, to not fall behind on the harvesting schedule. Working on land just treated was the hardest; the irritation of the eyes strongest. I got rashes on my hands from touching the soil, vegetables, and fruit with my bare skin. The common practice is to apply pesticides on a portion of the farm while farmworkers work on another. But even when they applied chemicals two or three fields away, the wind brought them to us."

The Worker Protection Standard for agriculture is designed to protect the two million agricultural workers and pesticide handlers. For greenhouse workers, entry is restricted anywhere from two hours after application if mechanical ventilation systems are in place, to twenty-four hours in structures with no ventilation.[46] The restricted-entry interval

43. Arthur Grube et al., *Pesticides Industry Sales and Usage: 2006 and 2007 Market Estimates*, US EPA, February 2011, http://www.epa.gov/opp00001/pestsales/07pestsales/market_estimates2007.pdf. This total includes all pesticides (herbicides, insecticides, miticides, fungicides, nematicide, fumigants, wood preservatives, and chemical biocides) used in agriculture, industry, commercial, government, homes and gardens. I excluded chlorine/hypochlorites used in water treatment, an additional 2.6 billion pounds. I used the most recent 2007 figures.

44. Marvin J. Levine, *Pesticides: A Toxic Bomb in Our Midst* (Westport, CT: Greenwood Publishing Group, 2007).

45. Arthur Grube et al., "Pesticides Industry Sales and Usage: 2006 and 2007 Market Estimates," US EPA, February 2011, http://www.epa.gov/opp00001/pestsales/07pestsales/market_estimates2007.pdf.

46. "How To Comply with the Worker Protection Standard for Agricultural Pesticides: What Employers Need to Know," US EPA, 2005, https://www.epa.gov/sites/production/files/2015-06/documents/epa-735-b-05-002.pdf. These are minimum standards. Each state or local governments can issue additional requirements.

on fields and orchards is dependent on the time interval indicated on the pesticide label.[47]

She looks over at her son Danny sitting near the entrance as he steadily adds soil and seeds to large cell packs. "I want limited exposure to chemicals for my family. My son became sick with cancer; leukemia. Thank God he survived, but his pancreas is compromised. He is now diabetic."

"Do you think his exposure to chemicals compromised his health?" Rain hits the plastic, first slow then with a ferocity drowning out the accordions and horns in the ranchera music.

"I imagine . . ." she stops speaking, as though building up the courage to say what comes next. "Yes, I took him with me to the fields so he'd learn how to work. Mostly to strawberry fields in Oxnard, California, where we lived for twelve years."

"I wanted him to experience firsthand how difficult life is for a farmworker," Nelida goes on, "so he'd pay more attention to his studies at school." The rain stops as if commanded.

I live near the fields Nelida and her son harvested. I've watched the chemical fog settle upon the delicate berries.

American farmers collectively spray 144 million gallons of chemical pesticides on cropland in one year.[48] Weightless droplets scatter with slight winds and updrafts. Each micro-droplet is anywhere between two and sixteen microns in diameter, smaller than a particle of dust. Half the poisonous mist lands on its intended target, and half drifts away from the fields.

Due to the inevitable nature of chemical drift, the USDA organic certification allows pesticide residues of up to 5 percent of the EPA tol-

---

47. Ibid.

48. Over 17,000 pesticide products are registered in the United States containing 800 active ingredients. The EPA registers pesticides based on test results provided by the registrant, the producer of the chemical product. Toxicology testing on laboratory animals is required for each single active ingredient even though most formulas are a combination of substances.

erance level.[49] When higher chemical residue is suspect, samples of soil, water, seeds, waste, and plants are tested. Five percent of organic food producers are tested on an annual basis, a rate five times higher than the number of household and businesses audited by the IRS.[50]

Strawberries are a permanent fixture on the Dirty Dozen list, an annual rating published by the Environmental Working Group (EWG).[51] The EWG analyzes samples of washed and peeled produce for pesticide residue. Scientists from Pesticide Action Network found fifty-three different residues on the popular berry, nine identified as known or probable carcinogens.[52] A common practice for strawberry crops is to spray fumigants like methyl bromide onto raised beds of soil, and then cover them with taut sheets of white plastic. Fumigants are among the most hazardous drift-prone pesticides. In California alone, fifty million pounds of fumigants are sprayed, most destined for a strawberry field.[53]

In the rain letup, we take the opportunity to move outside to her three-acre plot at Viva Farms. She farms an additional two acres of leased land in another location in Mt. Vernon. The ground is too muddy to walk the distance to her fields, so instead we drive. Once across, we leave the car in an empty parking lot of the Viva Farms produce stand.

---

49. For further information on how the EPA sets tolerance levels, visit http://www.epa.gov/pesticides/factsheets/stprf.htm.

50. Inspection and testing regulations of USDA organic certified foods are outlined in 7 CFR 205.603, found at https://www.law.cornell.edu/cfr/text/7/205.603.

51. "EWG's 2014 Shopper's Guide to Pesticides in Produce™," EWG, May 23, 2014, https://www.ewg.org/foodnews/dirty_dozen_list.php.

52. Leah Zerbe, "The Dark Side Of Strawberries: Are your berries harboring this unhealthy secret?," Prevention, April 23, 2013, http://www.prevention.com/food/healthy-eating-tips/strawberries-contain-large-amounts-chemicals-and-pesticides. Scientists with the Pesticide Action Network analyzed USDA data. In addition to the nine carcinogens, twenty-four are suspected hormone disruptors, eleven neurotoxins, twelve developmental or reproductive toxins, and nineteen honeybee toxins. Traces of fungicides captan and pyraclostrobin turned up on more than half of strawberry samples tested.

53. Paul Towers, "Strawberry Fumigant Pesticides Still Widely Used in California," Pesticide Action Network, June 19, 2013, http://www.panna.org/strawberry-fumigant-pesticides-still-widely-used-california. California grows 90 percent of US strawberries. US strawberries command 29 percent (2012) of the world market, the largest producer.

Closed now, it is a bustling marketplace in the summer and fall. At the stand, Nelida sells berries, vegetables, and homemade tamales stuffed with Swiss chard, kale, and cheese.

I follow in her footsteps down the outer edge of the field. Drip lines stretch along the crop rows. "How often do you need to irrigate?"

"Twice a season, depending on the wind and the heat. The water table is so high even lettuce and strawberries with short roots can reach it."

The water table below Nelida's farm is four to six inches below the surface in the wet season. This allows for the plants to be sub-irrigated by natural moisture. In the dry season the water table drops to twenty feet but is replenished with rain and snowmelt in time for the next growing season.

Alpine glaciers are integral to the Skagit River watershed here. The North Cascades range is home to 300 glaciers covering 62,000 acres.[54] These frozen reservoirs of fresh water cling to the stone and fill the cavities between mountains. The warmth of summer melts 230 billion gallons of that glacial snow, replenishing sinuous rivers and streams.

In recent years, early springs combined with more rain in the winter mean less summer runoff, according to the North Cascade Glacier Climate Project. They found a 25 percent decline in glacial area and volume, resulting in a 27 percent decline in summer streamflow compared to 1946. Two-thirds of the glaciers will not survive the end of this century. Glaciers have already disappeared, and if warmer temperatures continue as predicted, more will follow.[55]

Stalks of swiss chard left over from last year's crop outline the path. "When does your season begin?" I ask Nelida.

---

54. "Glaciers / Glacial Features," US National Park Service, https://www.nps.gov/noca/learn/nature/glaciers.htm. Washington is the second most glaciated state. Alaska is the first.

55. Mauri S. Pelto, "Impact of Climate Change on North Cascade Alpine Glaciers, and Alpine Runoff," *Northwest Science* 82, no. 1 (2008): 65–75. The North Cascade Glacier Climate Project (NCGCP) has been monitoring the alpine glaciers for more than three decades. Forty-seven glaciers are monitored as well as analyzed from the USDA Snow Course, SNOTEL data from eight stations and USGS runoff records. According to climate models in the Pacific Northwest, temperatures are expected to increase 1.7–2.8°C. Thank you to Mauri Pelto for reviewing this section for accuracy.

"The planting period is from May to October. I extend my season by planting early, in mid-March and lengthen it by growing crops suitable for the fall. I am waiting for five consecutive days of no rain. Soon after that, I'll disc the soil and add compost."

She continues, "I protect the sprouts from the cold with tents of plastic about two feet tall. The miniature hoop house speeds up the growing process, since plants grow slow in cold weather. I reuse the plastic for several seasons."

Metal hoops covered with plastic or fabric are sprouting on farms throughout the country.[56] Hoop houses, also called high tunnels, are warmed by trapped heat from the sun. The growth of lettuce greens and ripening of dainty strawberries are accelerated within the curved microclimate. The warm air lengthens the growing season; lettuce and tomatoes are able to grow in the snowy winter or soggy spring.

Evapotranspiration (ET) is water lost to the atmosphere from the ground and plants. Under plastic, fabric and glass enclosures, the ET drops 60–85 percent.[57]

A blueberry patch marks the end of her land. I'm careful to stay clear of the water pooling on the soggy soil, "How do you manage too much water?"

"I use different soil types to my advantage. Areas with sandy soil drain quickly. In those areas, I grow radishes. Other areas where the soil

56. Ted Blomgren and Tracy Frisch, "High Tunnels: Using Low-Cost Technology to Increase Yields Improve Quality and Extend the Season," University of Vermont Center for Sustainable Agriculture, May 2007, https://www.uvm.edu/~susagctr/resources/HighTunnels.pdf. Polyvinyl chloride (PVC) pipes are used as a low cost alternative to metal hoops. Hazardous organochlorine chemicals are released in large quantities into the air, water and soil both during its production and incineration (due to the chemical composition of PVC, recycling ranges from difficult to impossible).

57. Peter Tipis Ole Mpusia, "Comparison of Water Consumption between Greenhouse and Outdoor Cultivation," International Institute for Geo-informtation Science and Earth Observation, 2006, https://pdfs.semanticscholar.org/74ac/6a9733f986690e77626978fdc31759627707.pdf. The water saving is about 20–25 percent more than a drip irrigated open field and even higher when compared to a sprinkler or flood irrigated area.

stays moist longer, I grow plants like kale and chard. I don't plant in areas prone to flooding or pooled water because there is a higher chance of disease spreading, and the roots will rot. I know my seasons and my soil."

I bend down to break off a dried flower from the stem. I examine the stiff petals, the memory of its once bright color hidden, "How do you manage pests without the aid of chemical pesticides?"

"I don't have many problems. I plant flowers along the rows to attract beneficial insects. If I do get an infestation, it's confined to that one fruit or vegetable crop. Loss is minimized with a variety of crops. One season, pests attacked my broccoli. I mixed dishwashing soap, cooking oil, and water, and sprayed it on the infected plants. It worked."

The rain shifts from a drizzle to a steady downpour. On the return trip up the path, I keep up with her brisk pace. "What is your goal for the future?"

"My plan is to purchase land to farm and build a small house here in Mt. Vernon. Right now I'm looking at five acres for $180,000. I need a location with great visibility for a farm stand." When she smiles, her eyes disappear into squints. In a more serious tone she adds, "And I will help others in similar situations start their organic farms."

We drive back to the hoop house in silence.

In the quiet, I remember another car ride. It began in the translucent black before dawn in Oxnard and ended 200 miles away in Delano, California in the summer of 1988. My father, mother, younger sisters, and I sat under the feeble shade of a white canopy tent with 3,000 others, mostly farmworkers. We gathered to pray for the health of Cesar Chavez, who co-founded the United Farm Workers Union with Dolores Huerta. He fasted twenty-nine days to draw attention to pesticide use on the fields that he understood caused birth defects and cancer among farmworker children. His action was bold, like the color red.

Nelida's boldness comes in the form of her organic farm, growing food without chemicals, sowing seeds with her son. Against all odds, she has become a farmer. Each harvest a victory.

Nelida's Cheese, Swiss Chard, and Kale Tamales

Makes 10 servings, about 20 tamales

60 minutes to prepare (soak the corn husks first)

60–80 minutes to cook

All great tamale makers (*tamaleros*) have no written recipe. Their cookbook is visceral; they know how much ingredients to use by the look, feel, and taste. When I asked Nelida for her tamale recipe, she said, "Chop up some chard, kale, garlic . . . add a little bit of grated cheese and add it all to the *masa*."

For a tamale maker, these directions are sufficient. For me, not so much. I asked friends who I consider excellent *tamaleros* to help me translate. Their tips proved helpful, but everyone I asked used *masa preparada*: prepared cornmeal dough with *manteca*—lots and lots of lard.

I tried making the masa from scratch. I didn't want lard or GMO corn in my tamale recipe. Instead, I used Bob's Red Mill Masa Harina mixed with vegetable broth and olive oil. To my delight, the tamales were moist, delectable, and simple.

But the real test was if my mom liked them. My mother is rarely satisfied with a tamale, always complaining that the masa is too dry, flavorless, or *masudo*, a tamale with too much masa.

After the first bite, she declared it the best tamale she ever tasted. I hope you feel the same.

Ingredients

1 package corn husks

FOR THE FILLING:

2 tablespoons organic olive oil
1 medium head of organic garlic
1 large bunch organic swiss chard
1 large bunch organic kale
1 pound organic Monterey Jack cheese*
1 tablespoon salt

**Swap the cheese with a non-dairy substitute or hold the cheese altogether for a vegan tamale.*

FILLING VARIATION (*in addition to the ingredients listed for the filling*):

½ cup toasted pine nuts
Swap half the Monterey Jack with Parmigiano-Reggiano

FOR THE MASA (*corn meal dough*):

4½ cups organic/non-GMO Masa Harina (Bob's Red Mill brand is non-GMO)
3 cups organic vegetable broth
¼ cup organic olive oil
2 teaspoons salt

FOR THE CHILE SAUCE:

4 tablespoons organic olive oil
1 teaspoon organic all-purpose flour
1 tablespoon organic powder chile
½ teaspoon organic garlic powder
¼ teaspoon salt

Directions

1. Soak the corn husks in a large bowl/pot of warm water. This also works in the kitchen sink. Always do this step first to give the corn husks enough time to soften. After 45 (or until pliable) minutes take out of the water and pat dry. Water plants with the leftover water.
2. Chop the garlic, kale, and swiss chard. Sauté together in olive oil until the greens are just wilted. Put aside. For the chili sauce, heat olive oil on low flame in a medium pan. Combine remaining ingredients in a small bowl. Add dry ingredients to the oil and mix with a wooden spoon continuously for 2–3 minutes. Remove from flame and add the chard and kale mixture to the chili sauce.
3. Grate cheese and put aside. Monterey Jack is always a good choice for tamales, but experiment with your favorite cheese. Parmigiano-Reggiano mixed in with the Monterey Jack results in a rich buttery flavor.
4. Toast (optional) pine nuts on the stove top in a dry pan. I use a cast iron skillet. Pine nuts toast quickly, in about 3–5 minutes. Stir often until fragrant and golden brown. Transfer pine nuts immediately into a bowl to keep from burning.
5. Combine the ingredients for the masa in a large bowl. The consistency should be like chocolate chip cookie dough. Add more harina or broth as needed.
6. Open a corn husk and place in the palm of one hand. If corn husks are torn you can overlap two. In one hand hold the husk lengthwise and with the other spread 1½ generous tablespoons of masa. You can use anything to spread it; I personally prefer the back of the spoon. Spread the masa in the center area. Leaving about a ¾ to 1 inch margin on the bottom, but you can spread the masa all the way to the top edge. (You will need this

margin when folding the husk.) You will quickly learn there is no best way to do this. Every tamalera has his/her own style to spread.

7. Add 1 heaping tablespoon of the sautéed greens, and 2 tablespoons cheese. If you have pine nuts, sprinkle on top of the cheese.
8. Fold the husk around the filling. Wrap the sides first (like you do a burrito) and fold the bottom up. If your husk doesn't stay closed you can tear thin ribbons of husk to use as ties.
9. Stack tamales upright in an 8-quart steamer with a lid. If you don't have a steamer, get creative. You can place a steamer basket in a pan, use a canner, or do anything that lifts the tamales above the water. The steaming time varies. A small batch of tamales will take an hour, give or take. I start checking mine before the hour. (An over-steamed tamale is the *worst*!). Be sure to check your water level in the steamer too. When they look done, remove one tamale with tongs to check if the dough is thoroughly cooked. Just like a cupcake, cooked tamales have no wet dough and the husks will peel off easily.
10. To serve, peal off husk and top with a spoonful of green salsa. To make your own, see the tomatillo salsa recipe on page 106.

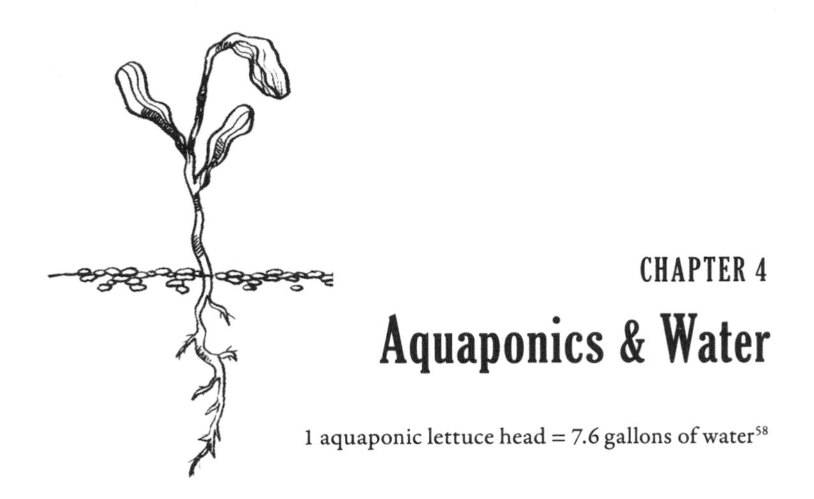

CHAPTER 4

Aquaponics & Water

1 aquaponic lettuce head = 7.6 gallons of water[58]

SUSTAINABLE FARMS RAISE a diversity of food. It's why I'm not too concerned when farmer Ben Godfrey tells me at the start of our interview, "We don't have any pigs at the moment," the planned topic of discussion.[59] Ben, owner of Sand Creek Farm in the Texas Plain, lists the many hats he wears: holistic-managed dairy farmer, cattleman, cheese maker, organic vegetable grower, horse rancher, and aquaponic farmer. I stop him at aquaponics. I am intrigued to understand how growing food in water fertilized by fish fits into the larger picture of a sustainable farm.

We walk toward a row of hoop houses, erected on a parcel of the 170 acres of Texas pasture and fields. Within minutes of being outside, we are damp. A cloudless sky offers no respite from a blazing August sun. Sweat runs down from the rim of Ben's cowboy hat; perspiration soaks his long-sleeved collar shirt. I'm reluctant to step inside the hoop house. I imagine it will be stifling inside the plastic structure.

"It would be hotter in here if we left all the plastic on," Ben says in response to my surprise at how much cooler it is inside the plastic. "These plants are 47 percent more shaded." A screen, like the kind used on a screen door, covers the ceiling and two sides. I look up from within the

58. "Water Usage in Recirculating Farms," Recirculating Farms Coalition, July 2011.
59. Ben Godfrey in discussion with the author, August 2014.

plastic to see black screens exposed overhead. "The heat dissipates out through the screen, so it doesn't get as hot. My plants are cooler and transpire less than crops grown outside."

In shallow pools of water, lettuce heads float on the surface in Styrofoam rafts. He tears off a piece of lettuce for me to try. The flavor is mild and sweet.

"Lettuce normally would be so bitter you can't stand it during this time of year. It is sweet because the roots are sitting in a body of water. The water temperature might be around eighty-five degrees, but the soil outside is one hundred." Ben lifts up one of the square rafts, exposing the stringy root systems hanging below. The roots look like long strands of corn silk.

The water footprint for a pound of traditionally grown lettuce is ten gallons of water. Lettuce and leafy greens demand a consistent water source. Under-watered lettuce goes to seed and turns bitter. In rainy climates, field greens require little irrigation during the sixty-five days between germination and harvest. But to grow lettuce in hot, dry temperatures, or areas with limited rainfall, irrigation is a must.

"Does aquaponics use less water than growing food in the ground?" I ask while I examine the roots.

"Ninety percent less water."

Ben bases this total from articles written about aquaponics. But few comprehensive studies are available on the actual water savings. One recent study conducted by researchers at John Hopkins University found more modest water savings between aquaponics and field-grown vegetables.

Researchers measured the water usage of the two most popular aquaponic grown crops, tomatoes and lettuce. They found tomatoes grown in an aquaponic system to consume less than the field-grown average, saving 48 percent. However, researchers found aquaponic grown lettuce requires 39 percent more water than lettuce grown in the field.[60]

"How much water is pumped through this system?" I notice the water level is at the 1,600-gallon line, indicated by embossed plastic numbers on the outside of the fish tank.

"We add water once, or twice a week. The rain tops the pools off too. Rain falls through the screen, but not much during this time of year." We look up at the big blue Texas sky beyond the screen.

The water source to replenish tanks is overwhelmingly *blue*, sourced from municipal drinking water sources and wells. In a survey of 809 aquaponic operators, 39 percent used rainwater. Water efficiency could be improved if captured rainfall were a more common source of water for aquaponics.[61]

"Do you ever change the water?" I ask.

"You don't need to. This is a closed-loop system."

Closed-loop systems recirculate the water from the fish tank into the grow beds in an endless loop. This is in contrast to an open-loop system where the water flows through the plant bed then is discharged.[62] Water can be recaptured and reused in an open-loop system to cut back

---

60. David C. Love, Michael S. Uhl, and Laura Genello, "Energy and water use of a small-scale raft aquaponics system in Baltimore, Maryland, United States," *Aquacultural Engineering* 68 (2015): 19–27. The study occurred over a twenty-four-month period at an aquaponic operation in Baltimore, Maryland. According to their data, they found it requires 13.5 gallons of water to produce one pound of edible crop. The water totals were higher to raise tilapia, at 39 gallons per pound of fish. The totals are based on the water necessary to "top off" due to evaporation, spillage, and leakage to a 10,000-gallons aquaponic system. The water footprint does not include the initial 10,000 gallons to fill a small-scale system.

61. Ibid.

62. The most recent survey was conducted in 1998: "Linking Hydroponics to a 880 Gallon Recycle Fish Rearing System," The Conservation Fund's Freshwater Institute,1998,http://www.aces.edu/dept/fisheries/education/documents/FWILinkingAquaponicsto880gRAS.pdf.

on water usage, but the cost of implementing recycling is a barrier for small soilless system operators like aquaponics and hydropnics.[63]

"What is the biggest difference between aquaponics and hydroponics?" There are 1,500 hydroponic operations out of 2.1 million farms.[64]

"Aquaponics is raising vegetables in fish water," he says. "With hydroponics, you add your nutrients and test the water a whole lot. You need to work hard to make hydroponic vegetables grow organically. But there is a growing demand for organic hydroponic."

No standards exist for organic hydroponic or aquaponic. The National Organic Standards Board (NOSB) recommended the prohibition of soilless agriculture for organic certification due to the absence of organic matter in the non-soil media of gravel, peat, pumice, and water. Despite the recommendation from the NOSB, the USDA's National Organic Program in 2014 opened the door to organic hydroponics, however it offered no guidelines or rules. Mexico, Canada, and Holland grow most of the organic certified hydroponics sold in the US. All three nations prohibit labeling of soilless agriculture sold in their own countries as organic.[65]

---

63. Howard M. Resh, *Hydroponic Food Production: A Definitive Guidebook for the Advanced Home Gardener and the Commercial Hydroponic Grower* (Baton Rouge: CRC Press, 2012). True hydroponics is water culture, but the definition has grown to include all non-soil mediums or soilless culture to grow plants. Examples of soilless-growing medias include gravel, peat, sawdust, pumice, and rice hulls. The common shortcoming of all forms of hydroponics and soilless culture is the necessity to add all the essential nutrients and minerals for plant growth.

64. "Hydroponic Crop Farming in the US: Market Research Report," IBISWorld, January 2016, https://www.ibisworld.com/industry/hydroponic-crop-farming.html. Hydroponics is expected to grow 3.3 percent between 2015 and 2020.

65. "Organic? USDA Hydroponic and Aquaponic Task Force," *Truthout*, March 18, 2015, http://www.truth-out.org/speakout/item/29736-is-hydroponics-organic. The NOSB position toward hydroponics is shared by several US organic certifying agencies as well as most countries, including Mexico, Canada and twenty-four European nations. Despite the recommendation from the NOSB, the USDA's National Organic Program in 2014 opened the door to organic hydroponic, however, offered no guidelines or rules.

"You don't need to add any nutrients to the water?" I ask, peering down into the opaque water.

"In aquaponics, the fish fertilize the water for you. See the worm-like things?" He points to squiggles floating on the surface of the water. "When I first started, I thought I'd bought wormy fish. I even bought a vacuum to suck the worms out. What I thought was worms was the fish manure, the fertilizer." Ben laughs at the memory. "I don't sample my water like they do in hydroponics. I just need to take good care of my fish and give them good quality feed."

"Where are the fish?" I try to catch a glimpse between the lettuce plants.

"The fish aren't in the pools. They'd eat my plants if they were." He leads me to a circular plastic barrel connected to a raised narrow pool. Inside the barrel the water is a rust color. The 400 pounds of tilapia is recognizable only as dark shadows beneath the water surface.

"Are most aquaponics organic?" I ask.

"Aquaponics is organic by default. The fish keep you honest. Chemicals would kill the fish."

Ben ushers me into the second of three hoop houses growing Asian greens. Small bouquets of mustard, mizuna, and bok choy sprout together in each water nested pot.

Spiders cling to elaborate webs near the tanks.

"We encourage those," Ben says, pointing out several webs spun in each corner. "See that grasshopper?" He points to a neon-yellow grasshopper just beyond the screen wall. "He wants to get in here and eat my plants. If he gets inside, these spiders will do their best to make a meal of a meaty grasshopper."

Aquaponics is a hybrid of hydroponics and aquaculture—fish farming—Ben explains. "In high-density aquaculture, plants were introduced to act as a natural filtration system. Without the plants, the water gets out of balance with too much ammonia or nitrates from the fish waste." The cultivation of plants alongside fish has been traced back to 1000 AD, when it was a practice of the Aztecs in what is now Mexico City.[66]

"Can the land absorb the excess nutrients produced by aquaponics?" I ask. Excess nutrients from animal husbandry is a concern as one of the top polluters of America's streams and rivers.

"Easily, even with the high-density aquaponics. Fish manure is a great nutrient. I spread the manure on the grass where my kids play. Aquaponics waste runoff is negligible because they're little fish. The accumulated waste is nothing in comparison to a cattle feedlot."[67]

We leave the shade of the hoop house. The pasture is as wide open as the sky. Few trees dot the landscape.

"Do you consider aquaponics a 'sustainable' agricultural model?" I ask.

He pauses to collect his thoughts. "I hesitate to use the word sustainable when describing aquaponics. Aquaponics will never be as sustainable as growing in dirt. My cattle eat from the pasture. The soil receives nutrients from the cover crops, and grazing cows trampling their own manure into the soil. But on a farm like ours, aquaponics and fields complement each other."

"How?"

"During the right season for those crops I grow in the field. But not many vegetables grow in the dry summer months, and cows produce hardly any milk during this time of year. Our primary income in the summer months is aquaponics."

"Aquaponics financially supports your sustainable farming during the off-season?"

---

66. Juanita Boutwell, "Aztecs' Aquaponics Revamped," *Napa Valley Register*, December 15, 2007.

67. See "Chapter 5: Seafood & Water" for more information on the impact of waste from aquaculture on water systems.

"Aquaponics is not sustainable like the pioneer-style farming I practice three-quarters of the year, but it is an important income stream."

The lettuce floating on Styrofoam rafts on a small slice of Ben's sprawling acres helps keep this farm afloat. Diverse income streams are as important to the vibrancy of sustainable farming as healthy soil.

Tofu over Sautéed Asian Greens

Makes 4 servings

15 minutes to prepare

7 minutes to cook

This recipe is inspired by Ben's Asian green bouquets of bok choy, mizuna, and mustard floating on square rafts. The recipe is just as good with spinach alone.

Ingredients

- 2½ ounce mixture of organic Asian greens (bok choy, mustard, mizuna, and spinach)
- 1 pound organic tofu (firm)
- ½ cup organic soy sauce
- 1 tablespoon organic Asian sesame oil
- 3 teaspoons organic dark brown sugar
- 3 teaspoons peeled and grated organic fresh ginger
- 2–4 organic garlic cloves, minced
- ½ teaspoon organic hot sauce or dried hot red pepper flakes
- 2 tablespoons organic olive or coconut oil plus 2 tablespoons for sauté

Directions

1. Rinse Asian greens, drain and set aside. Stir together soy sauce, sesame oil, brown sugar, ginger, garlic, hot sauce (or red

pepper flakes), and oil in a glass casserole or pie plate. Use ½ the marinade for the tofu. Reserve the rest for the Asian greens.

2. Add tofu slices in one layer and marinate. Turn tofu over every couple of minutes, 8 minutes total.
3. Heat a lightly oiled, well-seasoned ridged grill pan (this can work in a skillet too) over medium heat until hot but not smoking. Lift tofu from marinade with a slotted spatula and grill (reserve extra marinade for Asian greens). Turn the tofu over once carefully with a spatula, until grill marks appear and tofu is heated through, about 4–6 minutes for both sides.
4. Sauté greens in a large skillet in 2 tablespoons oil over medium heat. Toss greens with tongs until they begin to wilt. Add reserved marinade and sauté, tossing, until greens are barely wilted, about 1 minute. Divide among plates and add slices of grilled tofu on top. This also works over a serving of SRI and rice.

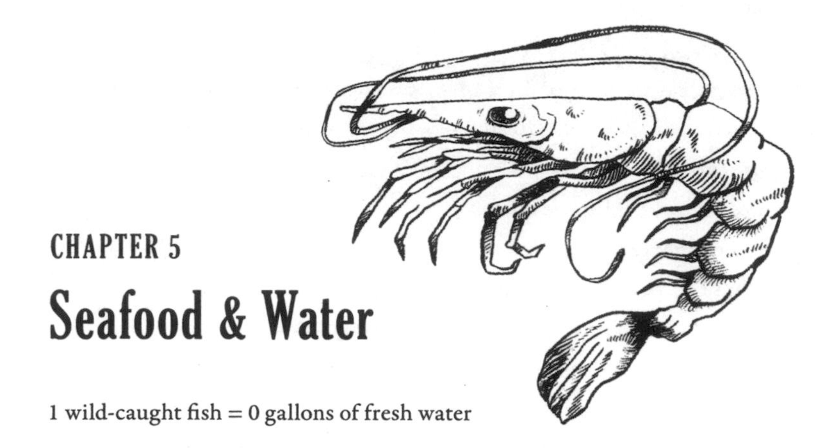

CHAPTER 5

Seafood & Water

1 wild-caught fish = 0 gallons of fresh water

"IN THE '70S, Winchester Bay was a thriving port when salmon fishing was robust on the Southern Oregon Coast. A hundred salmon boats were docked here," says Rick Goche, fisherman and owner of the Sacred Sea canned tuna label.[68] We both look out over the languid water, the quiet interrupted by the chime of the few sailboat masts.

"What changed?" I ask as we walk to his dry-docked boat in the shipyard. The boat is receiving needed repairs with help from his brother and grandson.

"Oregon resource managers convinced the public that fishermen were overfishing, but their explanation was bilgewater."

"Bilgewater?"

"Bullshit in seafaring vernacular." He laughs heartily. "Bilgewater is all the fish slime that comes out of the bottom of the boat." We climb the rungs of the ladder hanging down the side of the boat up to the ship's deck. "Make yourself at home." Rick points to a spot for me to sit near the stern.

"The hatcheries on the Columbia River were the biggest source of salmon on the West Coast. After the construction of dams, hatcheries were needed to mitigate the loss of natural runs. The Fish and Wildlife

68. Rick Goche in discussion with the author, June 2014.

Service took fingerlings and distributed them from hundreds of small creeks. Natural selection worked its magic and kept the stocks high. Then they changed the policy. They started to release older salmon, called smolts, from the hatcheries."

"How did that cause the collapse of the Oregon salmon fishery?" I ask. Fumes of primer and diesel overpower the scent of salty air.

"A Coho salmon takes one year to grow to the size of a smolt. While the fish are raised into smolts, they learned to expect food at the surface instead of hunting natural prey. When the smolts are released into a natural environment, they continued to find food at the surface, which made them easy prey. The birds decimated them."

"Why do you think they shifted to a one-hatchery model?"

"If you release salmon from only one hatchery, they return to the same hatchery, and you can count them and justify funding. The system collapsed after a few generations. A commercial fisherman hasn't caught a Coho salmon in Oregon in twenty years."

Pacific salmon are anadromous, starting their life in freshwater streams and rivers and migrating to the ocean. An adult spawner at the end of its life journeys upriver hundreds of miles to the stream of its birth. It reproduces once before it dies.

"Is there any discussion of reinstating the original hatchery model?" I ask.

"No, now the idea is to return to all-natural runs and natural spawning. But to bring salmon back, we need mitigation hatcheries."

"Why do salmon need hatcheries?"

"Dams," he answers. "Natural runs end with the construction of a dam on a waterway."

During the twentieth century, 75,000 dams were built on American Rivers. Dams powered the American industrial revolution and continue to protect human life and property from floods. Dams fostered the development of the Wild West. Water delivered from man-made reservoirs transformed deserts into fertile agricultural land. The Hoover Dam alone delivers irrigation to two million acres of cropland.[69]

"In California, salmon fishermen, in partnership with the state, transport the fish around irrigation pump areas and release them into San Francisco Bay. The waterways are so restricted and fouled up they don't have a choice."

Most rivers in the US remain fragmented. Complex ecosystems depend on free-flowing rivers. The halt of sediment naturally carried by rivers changes the shape of the American coastline, shrinking wetlands and stressing groundwater supplies. All fisheries suffer the stunting of rivers. Today, only 12 percent of the world's longest rivers run freely.

In the US, over 1,000 dams have been removed, with more slated for removal.[70] Meanwhile, worldwide, 1,500 new dams are currently under construction, including forty-six on China's Yangtze and a dozen more on the Amazon.[71]

"Salmon stocks would be stronger now if we had hatcheries, because the watersheds are cleaner today."

"Why?"

"Regulations. Regulations suck, but gosh they do some good things sometimes. Rivers aren't burning anymore."

The "burning" river polluted from industrial waste directly discharged into the river became a rallying cry for clean water activists in 1969. The Cuyahoga, which slices Cleveland into a distinct East and West side, was the most infamous burning river thanks to a story published by *Time* Magazine, but it was neither the first river to catch on fire nor the last. The frequent fires on the Chicago River became community

---

69. "Rivers at Risk: Dams and the Future of Freshwater Ecosystems," World Wildlife Fund, http://d2ouvy59p0dg6k.cloudfront.net/downloads/riversatriskfinalsummary.pdf.
70. "Frequently Asked Questions about Removing Dams," American Rivers, https://www.americanrivers.org/conservation-resources/river-restoration/removing-dams-faqs.
71. "Rivers at Risk," World Wildlife Fund.

spectacles. Chicagoans gathered on the moveable bridges to observe the river on fire like a fireworks display. Dirty rivers were a sign of progress.[72]

Cuyahoga River paved the way for the passage of the Clean Water Act (CWA), which became law in 1972 after an unsuccessful veto by President Nixon. The CWA regulates pollutant discharges into US wetlands, lakes, rivers, and streams and sets water-quality standards for "navigable," waters.[73] Agriculture, the leading polluter of American rivers, and lakes, is exempt from CWA rules.[74]

"I turned to the Dungeness crab market following the collapse of the salmon hatcheries. Crab is one of the most sustainable fisheries. You catch only males beyond breeding age and never the females; that's against the law. Females and breeding males can escape the cage because they are smaller in size. If a cage is lost, the lid closure is held closed with a biodegradable cotton so the crabs, even the non-breeding males, can escape."

Rick's brother Larry needs him in the engine room. I follow Rick inside as far as the dining area. I pause to appreciate the polished wood-panel walls. "Might as well have some nice digs. We're on this boat four months out of the year," Rick says after noticing my admiration for the craftsmanship.

The next room is a cabin with bunks and storage. I examine the beds and wonder how a man like Rick, with a build of a linebacker, squeezes himself into his allotted space.

We descend the narrow staircase to the lower deck, into the cavernous engine room. Larry is inside. They discuss an issue regarding hydraulics.

---

72. Hugh McDiarmid, Jr., "When Our Rivers Caught Fire," Michigan Environmental Council, July 2011, http://www.environmentalcouncil.org/priorities/article.php?x=264.
73. "Clean Water Act" (33 U.S.C §§ 1251 et seq), US EPA, 1972, https://www.law.cornell.edu/uscode/text/33/1251.
74. "Section 404 of the Clean Water Act: Exemptions to Permit Requirements," US EPA, https://www.epa.gov/cwa-404/exemptions-permit-requirements.

"Fishing is a lot more than just catching fish," I say as we climb up the stairs to the top deck.

"All fishermen need a broad skill set, but an albacore tuna fisherman even more so because you're 100–200 miles offshore," he says on the way back up the staircase. "The Coast Guard isn't going to come unless you're sinking. A tuna fisherman's skills have to include refrigeration, navigation, hydraulics, electrical, and mechanizing. *Then* you learn about fishing."

Back outside, everything is brighter. The cloud cover has burned off, leaving only the blue sky to contemplate. We sit down on top of the hinged door leading to the ship's hold.

"Why are you passionate about sustainable fishing?"

"I worked on a dragger as a young man. A dragger, or bottom-trawler, drags a wide net along the ocean bottom. The holes in the mesh are small enough to catch tens of thousands of little fish and a wide range of marine life. My job was to shovel them over the side along with the bycatch of bigger fish with no market value. These fish didn't swim off to continue with their happy life; they were all dead. The experience made me into the fisherman I am today."

"How does the dragger kill fish?"

"There are three ways to die: suffocation from silt clogging their gills, suffocation from being out of water, or suffocation from the weight of other fish."

Draggers also are responsible for nearly 80 percent of the global bycatch.[75] Half of global fishing production is caught with draggers.[76] The weighted nets dragged along the seafloor destroy fragile ecosystems.

75. The National Marine Fisheries Service defines bycatch as discarded catch of any living marine resource plus unobserved mortality due to a direct encounter with fishing gear.

76. Amanda Keledjian et al., "Wasted Catch: Unsolved Problems in US Fisheries," Oceana, March 2014, http://oceana.org/sites/default/files/reports/Bycatch_Report_FINAL.pdf.

One pass of a trawler can wipe away sea coral and sponges that took hundreds, in some cases thousands, of years to grow.[77]

"There are two sustainable methods to catch albacore tuna; *troll fishing* and *pole and line.* In troll fishing, big poles hang from the end of the boat with plastic lures attached to lines dragged along the surface of the water. Pole and line use live bait on handheld poles."

"Albacore swim near the surface?"

"Albacore is well out of range of our lures but every once in a while, they come up to start feeding. We count on it."

"Is bycatch eliminated when you fish near the surface?"

"Yes and no. Large commercial albacore fishing is often *longline* where hundreds or thousands of baited hooks drop below the surface. The hooks catch everything, like porpoise, whales, turtles, sharks, and seabirds."

Longlines from ships used in large-scale fishing operations can trail up to fifty miles behind the fishing vessel and reach below the surface twenty to thirty to forty feet. These longlines are prohibited in California, Oregon, and Washington, and regulated in the Atlantic and Hawaii. The South Pacific, the world's largest source of tuna, has no regulations.[78]

"How many tuna do you catch a day?"

"We try to average at least a ton a day. If we catch fourteen-pound fish, that is . . ." He quickly makes the calculation in his head. "143 fish a day."

Rick's grandson interrupts the interview to remind us of lunch. The three of us walk across the empty parking lot toward Double Ds on the Rocks, one of the few restaurants on the harbor.

---

77. "Position Statement: Bottom Trawling," World Wildlife Fund, 2007, http://www.wwf.se/source.php/1155231/WWF%20bottom%20trawling%20position%20statemest%20Nov%202007.pdf.

78. The Monterey Bay Aquarium Seafood Watch recommends longline be submerged to give clearance for marine life and to replace hooks with a circle hook allowing for easier release of unintended catches. Both measures significantly reduce bycatch.

"Tell me about Sacred Sea canned tuna," I ask on our walk. A *New York Times* article named Sacred Sea tuna a "Top Ten Pantry Essential."

"This is not your mother's tuna," Rick laughs. "I received an email from a mother who complained her kids won't eat the other brands after trying Sacred Sea. My tuna doesn't smell like anything you're used to."

"Why is your tuna different from the popular varieties?"

"For starters, the fish caught for large labels often die on the longline and go through the rigor mortis process on the hook. Once the fish dies, the oil begins to go rancid. Sacred Sea's entire fishing process from the sea to the can is engineered to preserve the flavorful and healthy oil. We pull them into the boat alive, one at a time. To enhance the flavor, we cut their throats, so they bleed out."

"Fish oil is what imparts the delicate flavor to fish. The correct freezing temperature, controlled thawing, and hand filleting is critical to keep the oil. These are all steps the big tuna labels skip. Take for instance the temperature. Our tuna is frozen at minus thirty degrees. The temperature is important because the enzymatic action that degrades the flesh is halted at minus twenty-eight degrees, and keeps the oils from migrating out of the fish. Big labels freeze at zero degrees. The reason they pack their tuna in vegetable oil, olive oil, and water is that all the fish oil leaks out. Our tuna is packed in fish oil made to cook with."

"It's not necessary to drain the liquid off your canned tuna?"

"No! It horrifies me to learn people drain the oil. Even some chefs throw out the liquid of our tuna, because that's what they're used to doing."

We sit at a corner table near the window. We are the only customers. "We catch smaller fish with troll fishing and pole and line."

"Does it matter if the fish are smaller?"

"Fish caught with longlines are bigger and older. Older albacore lose their oil content and taste drier, which explains why the big label tuna tastes like cat food. Besides improved flavor, younger fish are healthier because they are higher in Omega-3 and Omega-6."

The waitress hands us menus. I skip over the tuna fish salad on the menu made with big label tuna.

"Does the age of the fish affect mercury levels?"

"Absolutely. Older fish have accumulated environmental toxins from being on the food chain for a long time. The American Medical Association advises pregnant mothers against eating albacore tuna. Tuna caught with pole and line, or troll, are smaller, younger, and therefore haven't had enough time to accumulate mercury."

"What do you think about the advice of the American Medical Association?"

"Over-simplifying the issue does the consumer a disservice and hurts local fishermen. West Coast tuna is a healthy choice for pregnant women because of the Omega-3, Omega-6, and the balance of essential fatty acids, all perfect for brain development of the fetus."

Rick scans the menu. "The oysters and the shrimp are local." He points to the Oregon pink shrimp and Umpqua oysters listed on the menu. "The oysters are coming right from this bay, an appropriately applied aquaculture." Rick orders an Oregon pink shrimp cheese melt on rye bread with Double D's homemade chips. I order the Umpqua oyster basket named after the American Indian tribe indigenous to the Southern Oregon coastal region. It's also the name of the river that flows into Winchester Bay.

"What do you think about aquaculture?" I ask.

Aquaculture—fish farming—produces half of all fish consumed globally.[79] The totals are expected to surpass wild-caught fish within the decade.[80]

---

79. Christine M. Moffitt and Lubia Cajas-Cano, "Blue Growth: The 2014 FAO State of World Fisheries and Aquaculture," Food and Agriculture Organization of the United Nations, 2010, http://www.fao.org/docrep/013/i1820e/i1820e.pdf. The exact total is 46 percent.

80. "NOAA Fisheries," US National Oceanic and Atmospheric Administration, http://www.nmfs.noaa.gov/aquaculture/faqs/faq_aq_101.html.

"In my view, there are situations when aquaculture is appropriate and situations when it's just not. Every year in the US we eat a higher percentage of imported fish. Proponents of aquaculture see it as a means to reverse this trend."

American farm-raised fish, both marine and freshwater, represent only 7 percent of the national total of consumed seafood. Americans import 91 percent (fifteen billion pounds) of both farmed and wild seafood from overseas, the majority from China.[81]

United States fisheries are among the most regulated in the world. China along with other top seafood producers like India, Bangladesh and Vietnam, struggles with enforcement of environmental regulations. In China, 10,000 chemical plants are built along the rivers that flow into the China and Yellow Seas. Chemical spills into China's storied rivers are common.[82]

"Except for oysters and mussels, both filter feeders, aquaculture requires a food source. What is the origin of the fish food? You either take something from land, or you take from the ocean. The pellets fed to captive fish may or may not have chemicals or antibiotics added."

Carnivorous fish like salmon, striped bass, and tuna require fish meal and fish oil to thrive in captivity. Globally, one-third of all wild-caught fish is processed into fish meal.[83] The demand for wild fish to feed farmed fish takes a toll on marine ecosystems. For example, in 2015, the sardine population, a popular choice for fish feed along with anchovies, collapsed along the West Coast of the United States, prompting regu-

---

81. Paul Greenberg, interviewed by Terry Gross, *The Salt*, NPR, July 3, 2015, http://www.npr.org/sections/thesalt/2014/07/01/327248504/the-great-fish-swap-how-america-is-downgrading-its-seafood-supply.
82. "China's Rivers: Frontlines for Chemical Wastes," Worldwatch Institute, 2006, http://www.worldwatch.org/chinas-rivers-frontlines-chemical-wastes.
83. Rebecca J. Goldburg, Matthew S. Elliott, and Rosamond L. Naylor, "Marine Aquaculture in the United States: Environmental Impacts and Policy Options," Pew Oceans Commission, March 28, 2016, http://www.iatp.org/files/Marine_Aquaculture_in_the_United_States_Enviro.htm.

lators to cancel the sardine season. Starved sea lions washed up on the shore due to the reduction in sardine and anchovy populations.[84]

"The captive fish may or may not be in an area where there is enough flow to wash away their feces," he says just as our plates are served. While the amount of fish waste generated in an aquaculture operation is trivial in comparison to the accumulation of waste from a cattle feedlot, the environmental degradation to receiving waters is more detrimental. A Pew study found the fecal waste from a large salmon farm of 200,000 fish to be equivalent to the untreated sewage of 65,000 people. When fish waste is released untreated—as is the case with *Netpen* operations, fish held in net-like enclosures—fish waste flows directly into a body of water like a bay, estuary, lake or ocean.

"I'm reminded of a quote by author, Zora Neale Hurston," I say. "She wrote, 'all water is off on a journey unless it's in the sea, and it's homesick, and bound to make its way home someday.'"

Rick puts down his pink shrimp cheese melt without taking a bite. His demeanor turns serious, "Some of the apocalyptic projections I read about the impact of climate change on the oceans are terrifying. Climate change is felt in the ocean first and ripples throughout our global environment. Whatever we do, wherever we are, it ultimately impacts the rest of the planet."

The United Nations Intergovernmental Panel on Climate Change predicts a one meter sea level rise by 2100. The projection increases to two meters if the world's current rate of burning fossil fuels remains unchanged.[85] Under either circumstance, every continent in the world will change shape.

---

84. Peter Fimrite, "Sardine Population Collapses, Prompting Ban on Commercial Fishing," *San Francisco Chronicle*, April 14, 2015, http://www.sfgate.com/bayarea/article/Sardine-population-collapses-prompts-ban-on-6197380.php.
85. Ricarda Winkelmann et al., "Combustion of Available Fossil Fuel Resources Sufficient to Eliminate the Antarctic Ice Sheet," *Science Advances* 1, no.8 (2015), http://advances.sciencemag.org/content/1/8/e1500589.figures-only.

As the ocean grows, marine life totals will shrink. The ocean absorbs one-quarter of all CO_2 emissions. Scientists once believed this discovery to be good news. They thought the ocean absorbed CO_2 gases without any consequence. Now they understand CO_2 decreases the water's pH, causing ocean acidification. Ocean acidification hampers the ability of sea life to produce or maintain their shells. Much of our favorite seafood—oysters, clams, scallops, lobsters, shrimp, and crabs are vulnerable.

Oysters are the first victims to ocean acidification. The Northwest has lost billions of mollusks due to ocean acidification.[86]

Our vast oceans are what set Earth apart from every planet in our solar system. All life depends upon the water, and water is what may take life away. With sea level rise, species by species, square mile by square mile, will "return to the ocean," as Zora Neale Hurston wrote. But the story can be rewritten. It begins with the active engagement in our choices.

Change starts with our food.

86. Craig Welch, "Sea Change: Oysters Dying as Coast Is Hit Hard," *Seattle Times*, 2014, http://apps.seattletimes.com/reports/sea-change/2013/sep/11/oysters-hit-hard.

Pole and Line or Troll-Caught Tuna and Organic Gorgonzola Quesadillas

Makes 4 servings

15 minutes to prepare

2 minutes to cook (each pan of quesadillas)

Quesadillas are a food staple in my home. I add jalapeños, grilled bell peppers, turkey . . . but I never once considered adding tuna salad. Rick's youngest daughter created this recipe and insisted her reluctant father try it. They were so tasty Rick's son built two successful food carts in the Portland area selling them. (In Portland you can get one direct from Rick's son at Killa Dilla cart.) What makes these quesadillas amazing is the quality of tuna. Look for "pole and line" or "troll caught" packed in its own fish oil. It will indicate on the label.

Ingredients

4 organic flour tortillas (seek out a brand *without* palm oil)[87]

1 cup (¼ cup for each quesadilla) shredded or sliced organic Gorgonzola cheese or your favorite organic cheese (cheddar, mozzarella, pepper jack)*

A pat of organic butter or tablespoon of organic oil for the pan*

**Purchase dairy products from farms who practice a managed intensive rotational system (see "Chapter 9: Dairy & Water" for more information)*

87. See "Chapter 11: Chocolate & Water" for a discussion on palm oil.

FOR THE TUNA SALAD:

1 can of Sacred Sea tuna or similar brand
2–3 tablespoons organic mayonnaise
¼ teaspoon organic cumin
Capers (optional)
A capful of organic hickory smoke sauce of your choice (optional)

Directions

1. Mix together the tuna salad ingredients. Remember: DO NOT drain the fish oil if using Sacred Sea or a brand packed in fish oil.
2. On a medium flame, heat an oiled pan large enough to accommodate an open flour tortilla.
3. Smear a generous helping of tuna salad on one-half of the tortilla and sprinkle cheese on the other half. Fold the tortilla in half.
4. Fry the quesadilla slightly until the cheese melts and the tortilla gets a little crispy on both sides.

Wild-Caught Baked Salmon

Serving size depends on the size of the filet

15 minutes to prepare

60 minutes to cook per inch of filet thickness

Ingredients

Whole wild-caught salmon or filet

1 organic onion, sliced

Organic mayonnaise, enough to spread on the fish inside and out

1 teaspoon organic garlic powder

1 teaspoon salt

1 teaspoon organic pepper

1 organic lemon (optional)

Directions

1. Preheat the oven to 275 or 300°F.
2. Stuff the whole salmon with sliced onions or place onions on top of filet after step 4.
3. Slather mayonnaise all over the fish with your hands or a butter knife. Don't forget to spread on the inside of the fish cavity.
4. Season with garlic powder, salt, and pepper to taste.
5. Wrap the fish in foil, place on baking sheet, and put it in the oven. Bake an hour per inch of the thickness. For example, if the fish is 1½ inches thick, bake for 1 hour 30 minutes.
6. Squeeze lemon on top just before serving.

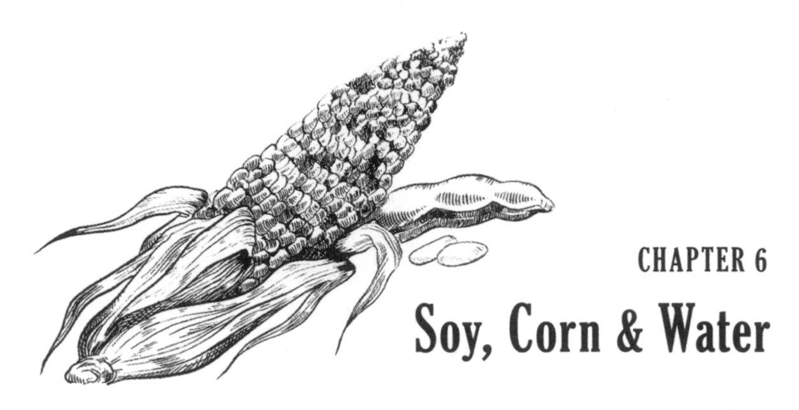

CHAPTER 6

Soy, Corn & Water

1 pound of corn = 146 gallons of water[88]

1 pound of soy = 224 gallons of water[89]

"PLANTS GROWN IN healthy soil need less water," says Alfred Farris, a Tennessee corn and soy farmer as he settles deep into his wingback chair. "Cover crop is the most important plant we grow, because it gives back to the land. At the end of the growing season we roll over the plants, creating a mulch about three inches thick, and plant right into it. The mulch combined with the cover crop keeps water on this farm."

Alfred with his wife Carney are no-till farmers.[90] According to the USDA Economic Research Service, no-till farming builds organic matter in the soil proven to retain higher levels of water. But organic matter is diminished with each application of chemical fertilizers and pesticides.

~

Organic soy and corn fields are a rarity in the US. In 2015, 94 percent of soybean and 89 percent of corn were grown from genetically engineered

88. "Product gallery," Water Footprint Network, http://waterfootprint.org/en/resources/interactive-tools/product-gallery.
89. Thomas Kostigen, *The Green Blue Book: The Simple Water-Savings Guide to Everything in Your Life* (Emmaus, PA: Rodale, 2010).
90. Albert Farris and Carney Farris in discussion with the author, August 2015.

(GE) seeds designed to be paired with herbicides.[91] Alfred and Carney's 470-acre farm is the only no-till, organic soy and corn farm east or west of the Mississippi. There is an upward trend of no-till acreage among the eight major crops over the past decade. Soy is the leading no-till crop with about 45 percent.[92] But unlike Alfred and Carney's Windy Acres Farm, these no-till farms are not organic.

"When did you begin growing corn and soy without chemicals?" I ask. Carney is the first to answer. "Many young people lived and worked on our previous farm during a ten-year period." She sits across her husband of sixty years. Barrettes tame her bobbed silver hair.

"These young people, including our children, were part of an environmental movement sparked by the book *Silent Spring*," says Alfred. In his Sunday best he looks more like a retired college professor than a farmer. "They asked us how we can claim to care for the creation that belongs to God with our chemical approach to farming. At first, I wasn't sure we could farm without chemicals. But we bit the bullet and began our long journey into organic farming, eventually adopting organic, no-till methods."

Published in 1962, *Silent Spring* cataloged the impact of chemicals on the environment and human health. The international bestseller led to the establishment of the EPA, Earth Day and the banning of DDT

91. Jorge Fernandez-Cornejo et al., "Genetically Engineered Crops in the United States," USDA Economic Research Service, February 2014, http://web.archive.org/web/20170404044049/https://www.ers.usda.gov/webdocs/publications/err162/43667_err162_summary.pdf. GE and GMO are often used interchangeably but they are not the same thing. GE can only occur with human intervention by transferring genes between otherwise sexually incompatible organisms. According to the USDA definition, GMO refers to any type of modification, from high tech genetic engineering to traditional cross-breeding that occurs naturally in nature. Sixteen GE plants are approved for American soil.

92. "USDA ERS—Crop & Livestock Practices: Soil Tillage and Crop Rotation," USDA, March 2016, http://www.ers.usda.gov/topics/farm-practices-management/crop-livestock-practices/soil-tillage-and-crop-rotation.aspx#.U1_tG_ldWSo. Based on 2006 figures, the most recent census data.

for domestic use in the US. Today, two and a half times more chemicals are sprayed on US cropland than in 1960, the increase mainly attributed to genetically engineered corn and soy crops.

~

We move outside. The farm surrounds the house on all sides. I've come to expect homes to be prominent fixtures on sustainable farms. When cared for, the land is a place where people want to stay, raising families alongside their crops.

We climb aboard the truck for the tour, leaving behind Carney's Prius with a *Stop Fracking* sticker affixed to the bumper. Our first stop is a fenced area of pasture near their house. The cows are British White cattle, an old heritage breed from England, dating back to Roman times.

"This breed has never been feedlot cattle. They get fat on grass," Alfred explains as we drive into the cattle paddock. The cows graze on the field of red clover uninterrupted by the truck.

"Are the animals part of your crop rotation?" I ask.

"Yes, three years of animals and three years of crops," says Alfred.

Alfred explains the sequence of cover crop rotation. They experiment with timing and sequences to promote the highest yields without the aid of fertilizers. The cover crop *is* the fertilizer, augmented at times with trace minerals and compost.

We watch the cows graze for a few moments in silence. Carney says in a whisper, "How they can convert grass into something ideal for the soil is magic."

Alfred pulls the truck over alongside the paddock fence. We walk toward the crimper, a smooth steel roller with shallow strips of metal attached in a chevron pattern. The crimper replaces the plow on a no-till farm.

We walk to the nearby field of soybeans. The crunch of mulch underfoot sounds like a bite of celery.

"This was rye." Alfred bends down to grab a handful of the dried plants in his hand. "The crimper rolled over the field, and soybeans were planted right into it. You can see we got some weeds, but there are plenty of beans growing out here even in this drought. Carney starts pulling weeds as we walk around the field. She is surprised by how easily the roots slip out of the ground.

"There is still a lot of moisture," she yells over to her husband.

Alfred walks toward her. "It's amazing given how dry it is."

I join them in pulling weeds. "See how long the root system is?" Carney asks me. "And feel how moist." I reach for the dangling roots in Carney's hands.

"Why don't you want weeds?"

"The soybeans next to the weeds are competing for water and nutrients. Mulch helps to suppress the weeds but not eliminate them."

In the middle of the field, the only sound is the buzzing and hissing of insects penetrating through the thick humidity.

"Are the yields higher for conventionally raised soybeans?"

"It's pretty close, and our input costs are a lot less. We're not buying all kinds of chemicals or GMO seeds."

Herbicide-resistant seeds, commonly known as GMO seeds, were professed to be an environmental breakthrough when first introduced in the 1990s. Glyphosate, the key ingredient in Roundup, was less toxic than its contemporaries, and required fewer applications to kill competing weeds without harming the intended crop. In the early years, this was true, and overall herbicide use waned. Soil erosion caused by tillage used for weed control was down too.

But weeds have built a resistance to the herbicides, spawning an aggressive strain of resistant superweeds. The Palmer Amaranth weed, for example, grows to be eight feet tall, with a sturdy stem that damages machinery.[93]

Half of all farmers surveyed in 2012 (the latest figures available), reported the presence of superweeds on their farms. In one year alone, the area infested with glyphosate-resistant weeds rose from 40.7 to 61.2 million acres, requiring increased applications of herbicides and tillage.[94] Overall, researchers estimate GMO crops are to blame for the 404 million pound increase of herbicides, a 7 percent increase over a fifteen-year period.[95]

Through the car window, Alfred points to a line of saplings planted along the border of their fields. "We planted hybrid chestnut and hazelnuts to provide wildlife habitat, shade for the cattle, and a buffer from the spray drift from our neighbors."

"Is cross-pollination with GMO plants a big concern?" Nature is insistent about reproduction. The wind, water, birds, and insects carry pollen from male plants and fertilize a female plant. A plant grown from an engineered seed in a laboratory is no exception.

"A big concern," they say in unison.

"During planting time, we watch our neighbors like a hawk. I write down the days they plant in my diary. I must be certain we stagger our planting so we won't be pollinating at the same time. We plant about a month later, and it costs us," says Alfred as he drives onto the town road.

There are no mechanisms in place to compensate non-GMO or organic farmers for economic loss due to delayed planting or cross-pol-

93. "List of Herbicide-Resistant Weeds by Herbicide Mode of Action," International Survey of Herbicide Resistant Weeds, http://weedscience.org/summary/moa.aspx?MOAID=12. One hundred fifty-one species of superweeds grow on United States crop acres, according to the International Survey of Herbicide-Resistant Weeds. Thirteen species are resistant to glyphosate.

94. Kent Fraser, "Glyphosate Resistant Weeds-Intensifying," Stratus Ag Research (blog), January 2013, http://www.stratusresearch.com/newsroom/glyphosate-resistant-weeds-intensifying.

95. "The Rise of Superweeds—and What to Do About It: Policy Brief," Union of Concerned Scientists, December 2013, http://www.ucsusa.org/sites/default/files/legacy/assets/documents/food_and_agriculture/rise-of-superweeds.pdf.

lination.[96] The USDA Advisory Committee on Biotechnology in the Twenty-First Century (AC21), recommends compensation modeled on existing crop insurance, but for now the burden belongs to the non-GMO farmers alone.

WELCOME TO ORLINDA, THE SUNNIEST SPOT IN TENNESSEE. I read the sign to mark the entrance of the town aloud. We pull off the road onto a field of corn.

In the field, Alfred reaches for an ear of corn. He peels off part of the husk and brushes away the silky fibers to expose the plump kernels. He offers me a bite. The fragrance of the corn is strong, like freshly mown grass. The kernels are sweet and juicy. Alfred and Carney take a nibble too.

"If we can get some rain on this crop, it will be fine," Alfred says mostly to Carney.

Buckwheat blooms with small clusters of delicate white petals on the adjoining field.

"We want something growing all the time," says Alfred. "The worst thing you can do is plow in the fall and leave the land bare through the winter. The rain will wash away the nutrients, and the water will evaporate or runoff without roots in the soil," says Alfred. Deep-rooted cover crops are found to reduce nutrient and pesticide run off by 50 percent or more. According to the most recent USDA Census of Agriculture, crop cover is planted on only 6 percent of farms. The total number drops further among farms larger than 200 acres to under 2 percent.

"Roots lead to healthy soil. Healthy soil keeps the water from running off or evaporating," adds Carney. On Windy Acres Farm the soil acts as a reservoir, saving water between the granules of dirt of the Farris' healthy land.

---

96. "Enhancing Coexistence: A Report of the AC21 to the Secretary of Agriculture," USDA Advisory Committee on Biotechnology and 21st Century Agriculture (AC21), 2012, http://www.usda.gov/documents/ac21_report-enhancing-coexistence.pdf.

Carney's Country Style Grits

Makes 2 full plates or 4 sides

5 minutes to prepare

10 minutes to cook

Corn Grits are a favorite of Carney and Alfred. They use their Golden Jubilee open-pollinated corn. The first time I made this recipe, I started with the corn kernels Carney sent me in the mail. I used a heavy duty blender to mill the grain. Corn grits are available in the grain or cereal section of your grocery store. Arrowhead Mills and Bob's Red Mill offer organic corn grits. When we purchase organic corn, we send a message to influential food corporations that there is a market for non-GMO corn.

Ingredients

- 2 cups filtered water (or 1 cup filtered water with 1 cup cream or creamy milk)*
- ½ cup organic or non-GMO grits
- ½ teaspoon salt (sea salt or mineral salt)
- 2 tablespoons organic butter
- ¼ cup shredded organic cheddar cheese (optional)

**Ratio of water to grits is usually 3:1 or 4:1 (adjust to suit to your liking)*

Directions

1. Combine water, salt, butter in a pan on high heat.
2. Add grits slowly to boiling water.
3. Whisk frequently till creamy (about 5 minutes).
4. Lower temperature and cover for an additional 5 minutes. You want the grits to have the consistency of cream of wheat, thick and creamy.
5. Stir in additional butter (about ½ tablespoon), cheese for rich flavor and serve.

CHAPTER 7

Eggs & Water

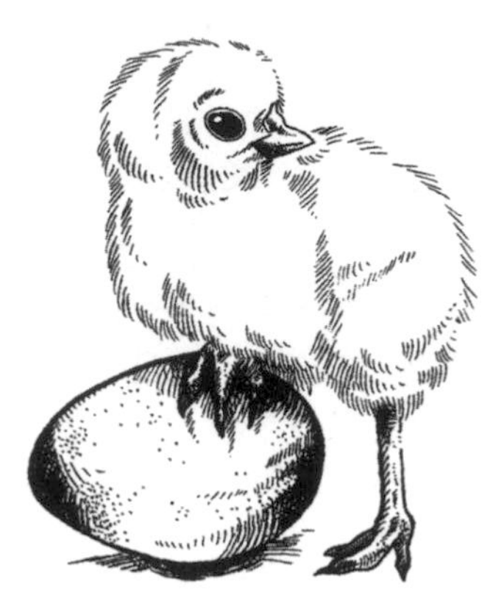

1 egg = 23 gallons of water[97]

1 dozen eggs = 276 gallons of water

THE AVERAGE ANNUAL individual American egg appetite (250 eggs per year) requires 6,000 gallons of fresh water. The largest share of water to produce eggs flows to the fields of grain. According to the USDA, chickens are a "major feed grain user." Chickens, the kind raised for meat and those raised for eggs, eat approximately one hundred billion pounds of feed a year.[98] My hunt for *green* eggs, defined as eggs grown with rain and moisture trapped in the soil, landed me in Elgin, Texas, home to the largest single-pastured egg operation in the United States with 25,000 hens and the first organic feed mill in the state.

"In the early days, my late father drove all over Texas picking up organic grains for his chickens," owner Rob Cunningham tells me as we stand inside the Coyote Creek Farm grain mill that smells like rising dough.[99] "It was difficult to find farmers growing organic grains. It wasn't that they didn't want to, they just didn't have a place to sell. But locating ingredients was too much wear and tear on him and his old

97. M. M. Mekonnen and A. Y. Hoekstra, "A Global Assessment of the Water Footprint of Farm Animal Products," *Ecosystems* 15, no.3: 401–415.
98. "American Egg Farming: How We Produce an Abundance of Affordable, Safe Food," United Egg, http://www.unitedegg.org/information/pdf/American_Egg_Farming.pdf.
99. Rob Cunningham in discussion with the author, August 2015.

blue truck, and he knew something had to change if he was to stay in business."

In America only 0.2 percent of soy and corn fields, the leading ingredients of livestock feed, are organic. The demand for organic feed outpaces the supply, causing livestock operations to seek sources from overseas, or to abandon organic farming altogether. But this sixty-acre farm with its cluster of gleaming feed silos and elevator stretching upward, shows us that the possibilities for reversing the trend of thirsty, chemically treated cropland are as endless as the big Texas sky.

Near the feed mixer, Rob flips the switch for corn. Corn kernels flow down the chute like a golden river. "We can mix 6,000 pounds of feed in this mixer at any given time."

"Where does the grain go from here?" I ask.

"We either send it into the mixer or outside to the elevators, the tall silver structures on top of the mill."

"Is this the standard way a feed mill works?"

"They all work the same," he says, leading me outside to examine the elevator conveying grain to the structure one hundred feet overhead. But this mill is far from ordinary. This mill is directly responsible for the conversion of 8,000 acres of American cropland from conventional to organic.

We leave the mill and walk up the path toward the barn. Two dogs lag behind. I follow Rob into a cordoned area. We are surrounded by pullets on all sides. "When they are chicks we can get 2,000 in here."

"How do the chicks arrive at the farm?"

"I like to say I pick up chicks in my wife's minivan."

I laugh on cue.

"We buy them from a hatchery here in Texas," Rob continues. "The van works great because it's climate-controlled. One hundred chicks come in a box the size of a milk crate. Every time I step on the brakes I hear 4,000 little feet scratching. It sounds like a loud rain stick."

We move back onto the path and walk toward the barn that houses the chicks. "We raise our chicks inside the barn because they can't yet regulate their own body temperature," Rob explains. "After three weeks, we move them outside into a temperature-controlled fenced-in area, a brooder yard, before they're moved onto the pasture."

Inside the structure, Rob's voice echoes in the hollow space. The chicks barely reach our ankles. They appear tinier near Rob's six-foot-eight frame. "The feed they eat is milled just a few minutes' walk up the road. That corn was just cracked a couple days ago. There is no fresher way to feed birds than how we're doing it." He squats down near a platter of feed on the barn floor and scoops a handful of cracked corn. A few chicks peck the kernels from his outstretched hand.

"How much pasture do chickens eat?"

"Chickens are herbivores. Thirty percent of their diet is from pasture, the rest is from feed. From the grass they get Omega-3s and other nutrients that come from grass alone. From the feed they get additional calcium, protein, carbohydrates. Ultimately the birds have free choice between feed and pasture. They intuitively know which nutrients their bodies lack."

Rob unlatches the gate of the white picket fence bordering the one hundred-year-old bungalow on the farm he shares with his wife and two teenage sons. It was his parents' home. Slumbering under the shade of a peach tree is a calf. "This is Jolene." He explains how she lost her mother. He squats down to scratch Jolene's belly after greeting her with the tender puckered talk usually reserved for babies.

"Is she named after the song?" I ask.

He answers with lyrics to Dolly Parton's famous song.

"How do the cattle fit into the pasture rotation?"

"We rotate the chickens behind the cows on a weekly basis. But in the summer, I can't keep the cattle on open pasture because they need access to shade. We have plans to set up more shade around the pasture.

In the meantime, the cattle can be found lounging under trees around the property."

Rotating two or more livestock in the same pasture is referred to as multi-species grazing. Multi-grazing is found to reduce parasites in animals, eliminating the need for deworming pharmaceuticals on farms that implement the practice. A parasite must complete its life cycle in the same species to survive. When larvae are eaten by a different species, they die. A study conducted by Oklahoma State University found a 75 percent drop in deworming treatments on animals raised in a multi-grazed operation.[100] One billion dollars is spent annually in the US on parasite control for cattle alone.[101]

We enter an old wooden carriage house with Jolene close behind. "One of the things my dad and I started doing years ago is to make teas for soil health. We brew our teas in here." He stands beside a cluster of fifty-five-gallon plastic drums. "We take a screen mesh, put it over the barrel, and add ten pounds of compost, worm castings, and organic molasses. With ten packs of compost, we brew 250 gallons of compost tea, enough to spray twenty acres. The tea fosters the same amount of organisms as if we spent thousands of dollars on compost to cover all sixty acres."

Jolene nudges Rob while he stands near the barrels of compost tea, knocking him off balance. Next she comes for me. "I've never seen this before," Rob nervously laughs while trying to contain her.

Rob calms down the 400-pound calf and continues my tour, "Since we started using the tea, the ground just soaks up every drop of rainfall. The soil is like a sponge. All the microorganisms increase the tilth, the pores in the soil that hold water. Because our soil absorbs every last bit of rain, we never need to irrigate, not even during the worst drought."

---

100. Anna Bennett, "Animal Welfare Approved Technical Advice Fact Sheet No. 4 Reducing the Risk of Internal Parasites," *Tech*, no. 4 (2009).
101. "Parasites and the Feedlot," *Beef Magazine*, August 1998, http://beefmagazine.com/mag/beef_parasites_feedlot.

Jolene jabs me off the path with her head and takes my place beside Rob. The three of us walk past areas of pasture where the Bermuda grass hugs the ground.

"The chickens were moved from the land two weeks earlier," Rob explains. "The birds haven't grazed in this patch of pasture for several weeks," says Rob. "You can see how quickly the pasture returns. Here we are in the middle of August, and there is plenty of green grass." The grass is tall and lush. "Enough to get us to the fall when it starts raining," he says just as Jolene hunches down and charges toward him, nearly knocking him over.

He steadies himself and continues the tour, now with a watchful eye on Jolene. "What we do is a textbook example of mob grazing but with chickens and rumens. They sample the grasses, scratch, drop their manure, leave their urine and are moved to a fresh pasture bi-monthly. In this system, the seeds are left in the ground and allowed to regerminate."

Mob grazing, also called holistic management or rotational grazing, replicates the natural movement of grazing animals in nature. I was first introduced to this farming technique on Maureen and Rob's Organic Valley dairy farm in upstate New York, but have seen variations of this method on every water-sustainable farm I've traveled to since.

The sound of clucking crescendos the closer we move to the hen house. Near the house, under the shade cloth, hens bathe in ash to control parasites. Rob raises his voice above the chicken banter, "We want them to exhibit as many natural behaviors as possible: eat grass, take dust baths, exercise, and socialize. Chickens can't do these things when cooped up in a barn twenty-four hours a day."

"Or confined to a battery cage," I add.

Ninety-five percent of hens spend their life in rows and columns of connected steel cages, called battery cages.[102] Four egg-laying hens

---

102. "American Egg Farming," United Egg. In the US, 95 percent of egg production is controlled by 235 farmers with flocks of 75,000 hens or more.

share residence in each cage, each with sixty-seven square inches of space on average (a smaller area than the size of standard notebook paper). Conveyor belts moving beneath the caged birds catch 222 million eggs and 33 million pounds of manure daily across the nation.[103] The point of destination of the eggs is clear; the destination for the manure is nebulous.

Michigan, Oregon, Ohio, and Washington State place restrictions on the size of cages.[104] Battery cages are outlawed in California. All eggs sold in the state of California must originate from hens with enough room to lie down, stand up, and extend their wings. But this doesn't necessarily mean that all eggs are now cage-free or pasture-raised in the Golden State. Instead, the battery cage is replaced with the "enriched colony cage." In this cage model, each bird is given a minimum of 116 square inches of space (equivalent to 1.33 sheets of notebook paper), enough room for the hen to spread her wings, but barely.[105] A conveyor belt moves underneath the slightly larger cage, catching the pharmaceutical tainted manure.

"What is the difference between pasture-raised eggs and cage-free?" I recall the labels printed on egg cartons found at my local grocery store.

The USDA offers no guidelines for cage-free or pasture-raised egg production. Cage-free birds are often housed in enclosed buildings with

---

103. The amount of manure is actually higher. This number considers the shrinkage of manure after the water is evaporated.

104. "Animal Industry Act 287.746," 1988, http://www.legislature.mi.gov/(S(zk3rmxiettouf0whp5fpecnz))/mileg.aspx?page=getObject&objectName=mcl-287-746. In the state of Michigan for example, the egg-laying hens must have access to at least 1.0 square foot of usable floor space.

105. Prop. 2 was passed in 2008 by a 65 percent margin and went into effect January 1, 2015. The state law requires farm animals to have enough room to lie down, stand up, extend their limbs and turn freely. The law applies to all eggs sold in the state even if produced out-of-state. The battery cage is replaced with the enriched colony cages, providing 116 square inches of space over the 67–86 square inch area for each bird in a battery cage.

large flocks, providing conditions for increased parasite and salmonella bacteria growth leading to increased pharmaceutical interventions.[106]

"Cage-free hens have room to walk around and nest, but it doesn't mean the birds live outdoors with access to pasture, and most don't. Pasture-raised is what you see here."

~

Inside, the hen house feels like a popular tavern on a Friday night. Chickens are perched along the sides of the walls up to the ceiling, socializing loudly with one another. Each house is built to accommodate 500 birds.

Rob places a speckled egg in my hand. The egg is still warm. "How often are eggs gathered?"

"Once in the morning and once after lunch. No egg is left in a nest box longer than twenty hours."

I wonder aloud how the birds are kept healthy at Coyote Creek. Growth hormones were banned from *all* poultry in 1950 but antibiotics and vaccinations are prevalent on conventional egg farm operations.[107]

"Every day we observe the chickens' behavior. One indication that there is a health problem is if their feed consumption drops. Healthy birds eat a quarter pound of feed a day. If a group of houses is not consuming that amount, we know they have a problem. In that case, we pick a sample and check for eye problems or parasites like lice under their wings. We examine the eyes and look through the feathers of ten

106. "Cage-Free vs. Battery-Cage Eggs," Humane Society, March 2016, http://www.humanesociety.org/issues/confinement_farm/facts/cage-free_vs_battery-cage.html.
107. "Chickens Do Not Receive Growth Hormones: So Why All the Confusion?," The Poultry Site, April 23, 2013, http://www.thepoultrysite.com/articles/2812/chickens-do-not-receive-growth-hormones-so-why-all-the-confusion. For a list of allowable vaccinations for organic certified livestock refer to 7 CFR 205.603, found at https://www.law.cornell.edu/cfr/text/7/205.603. Synthetic hormones are ineffective for poultry. In order for chemical (protein or steroid) hormones to be effective in poultry, hormones would need to be injected in the animal several times a day.

to fifteen chickens at random. If we find something, we use calendula oils, add organic apple cider vinegar, organic molasses, and salt to the drinking water for a little boost of electrolytes to aid in digestion and overall health."

Vaccinations and antibiotics to foster bird health are extraneous at Coyote Creek Farm. Birds have access to pasture, natural light, and ample space to stretch, scratch, and frolic as they choose.

We return Jolene to her favored spot under the peach tree inside Rob's fenced yard. I feel a wave of relief when he closes the gate, like when I close the door to my children's rooms at bedtime after a challenging day of parenting. I sense Rob feels the same.

A vast stretch of recently vacated pasture is near the mill. "This area was planted with winter rye, wheat, and oat the day the hen house was moved from the yard," Rob tells me. "As soon as any moisture hits that area, it will green right up." Today the patch is every shade of brown, baking under the summer sun.

"'The pasture is like breast milk,' my dad would often say. He compared the nutrition from a mother's food passed to her baby through her milk as a metaphor for the one-to-one connection between the grass and the chicken. Microorganisms feed the soil, soil feeds the grass, the nutrition from the grass passes into the eggs, and the animals feed you."

"There's another connection you missed," I say as we descend into the welcomed shade from the impressive mill above. He looks at me expectantly. "There is a one-to-one connection between the organic corn and grain farmer and this mill."

"Yes." He smiles broadly.

Green Eggs, Asparagus, and Spinach Quiche

Makes 8 servings

20 minutes to prepare

45 minutes to bake

Green refers to the color code of rainwater. Eggs produced from chickens raised on a diet of rain-fed pasture and grains are *green* eggs grown with natural rain. Once you find your green eggs, celebrate with the following quiche.

Consider the asparagus and spinach called for in this recipe as place holders. I change the vegetables to reflect what is in season and what I have in my vegetable bin. I use one to two vegetables. Be creative and modify to suit your favorite flavors and your organic and seasonal bounty.

Ingredients

6–8 fresh organic asparagus stalks
2 tablespoons organic olive oil
4 organic eggs, beaten*
1 cup organic milk*
1 tablespoon organic flour
½ bunch of fresh organic spinach
1 cup shredded cheese. Use your favorite cheese or a combination. I used Monterey Jack*
½ teaspoon salt
Fresh cracked organic pepper to taste

½ teaspoon organic nutmeg

Garnish with shredded organic parmesan cheese*

1 organic pie crust (For the pie crust I usually purchase an organic whole wheat crust. When I'm ambitious I make my own. I double the recipe so I can freeze a second pie crust for another time.)

**Choose carefully when purchasing animal products. Buy from farms that are practicing a managed grazing system such as Coyote Creek Farm's.*

Directions

1. Preheat oven to 375°F.
2. Slice the asparagus stalk diagonally. Sauté the asparagus with 1 tablespoon of olive oil. Add the spinach in the final few minutes.
3. Whisk eggs in a medium bowl. Add shredded cheese, flour, milk, salt, pepper, nutmeg, asparagus, and spinach. Incorporate together and pour into the pastry shell.
4. Place in the center of a cookie sheet. Bake for 45 minutes. If not done, check the quiche in 5 minute intervals until ready.
5. Let the quiche set for 5–10 minutes before serving. Shred parmesan cheese on top and serve.

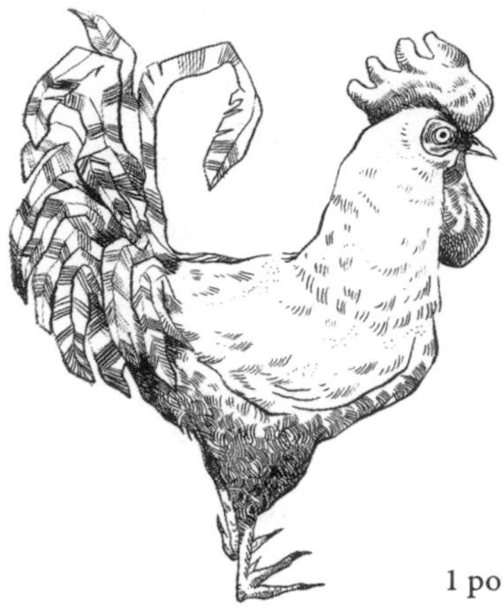

CHAPTER 8

Chicken & Water

1 pound of chicken = 468 gallons of water[108]

THE FIRST MEAL of roasted homegrown chicken Darinka Postal sat down at her kitchen table to eat ended in tears in the bathroom.[109] Darinka, a first-grade teacher, and her husband Paul, a lighting designer for Hollywood films, spent the previous year poring over books on raising chickens. Earlier in the day, their farm in Ojai, California, Funny Farms, had officially launched with the slaughter of their first flock.

They put into practice techniques they'd learned on YouTube. The slaughter of thirty chickens took from sunup to sundown, much longer than the video said it would. Darinka's reward at the end of the day was to prepare her first chicken for roasting.

"We'll have the freshest chicken available," she announced to Paul and her teenage daughter Chloe as she pulled the roasted bird out of the oven. It smelled glorious. The juices leaked out from the crackling golden skin.

She first suspected something was wrong as she worked her knife to negotiate the tough meat off the bone. Her first bite was chewy as a piece of chicken-flavored gum. Her second didn't improve. After her third bite, she fought back tears, grabbed the phone, ran to the bathroom, and shut

108. Kostigen, *The Green Blue Book*.

109. Darinka Postal and Paul Bly in discussion with the author, January 2011.

the door. Seated on the toilet, she dialed her farming mentor, Joel Salatin, 3,000 miles away, to ask him what she'd done wrong. Joel is a superstar farmer, familiar to the public from his appearances in the documentary *Food, Inc.* and Michael Pollan's book *The Omnivore's Dilemma*. He was not home to answer her call. It was Joel's daughter who tried to understand the incoherent syllables that squeezed out between sobs.

It was Paul who concluded, after a quick internet search, that the roasted meat was too fresh: chicken needs to sit at least a full twenty-four hours before the meat is ready to be cooked. Food too fresh to eat is unheard of in our modern food systems. Refrigerated semi trucks, warehouses, and grocery freezers work against the clock to keep food from spoiling.

Spoiled and unsold food is thrown away at every stop on the food-production chain. Between 30–50 percent of all food produced in the United States is wasted: wasted at the farm, the processing plant, supermarket, restaurant, and home kitchen.[110]

The average five-pound chicken requires 2,340 gallons of fresh water to raise, slaughter, and package, enough water to fill thirty bathtubs. Twenty-one million broilers—hens raised for meat—are slaughtered each day in the US alone, bringing the water footprint for our collective appetite to fifty billion gallons of fresh water per day.[111] Food in trash bins represents billions of gallons of wasted fresh water.

At Funny Farms, every chicken makes its way to a home refrigerator within eight hours. The total number of chickens processed is based on the total reserved in advance. Customers order by Saturday morning

---

110. Jonathan Bloom, *American Wasteland: How Americans Throw Away Nearly Half of Its Food* (Cambridge, Massachusetts: De Capo Lifelong Books, 2011).

111. "Livestock, Dairy, and Poultry Outlook: August 2013," USDA ERS, August 26, 2013, https://www.ers.usda.gov/publications/pub-details/?pubid=37524. Used projected annual totals for 2014. This total is the sum of multiplying the number of slaughtered hens per day (21,287,671 million) with the water footprint of the average five-pound chicken (2,340). The exact total is 49,813,150,684.931 gallons. I rounded up to 50 billion gallons.

(processing day) and pick up their chickens Saturday afternoon. Purchasing direct from the farmer eliminates waste in the conventional journey of food from farm to dinner plate.

"Why did you become a chicken farmer?" I ask Darinka. I am curious how a woman who had once been a Ralph Lauren executive, owner of a popular coffee house, and a first-grade teacher becomes a chicken farmer.

"I don't want my family to eat chicken that spends its life in a thick layer of its poop, inhaling the stench of ammonia," she says, referring to concentrated animal feeding operations (CAFOs) housing upwards of 125,000 birds under one roof.[112] "We want an alternative for ourselves and the ability to offer an alternative to our community," she explains.

I follow Darinka into a fragrant orchard of oranges. From this perspective, it's difficult to find any signs of a chicken farm: no barns, no sprawling hen houses are on this one-acre plot bordering the Ventura River. The only visible structure is a yurt in the distance.

"Where are the chickens?" I ask as I peer down the lines of orange trees. Darinka, whose smooth, pulled-back hair and subtle make-up give no indication she has been at work on the farm since 6:30 a.m., leads me to a three-foot-tall wooden box.

"These chicken houses are a Joel Salatin design," she says, as though we were discussing a piece of art.

The open-air roof of the chicken tractor is made from chicken wire on the 12×12-inch wooden crate. A continuous ballad of clucks rises from several dozen hens within as they move between a bucket of seed and pockets of newly sprouted grass. The floorless design allows the chickens to eat grass and insects directly from the land.

"Thirty percent of their diet comes from grass, the rest from organic feed," Darinka explains as we stare down at the young hens through the

---

112. Alan Sutton, Don Jones, and Katie Darr, "What is a CFO, CAFO?," Purdue University, July 2007, http://www.extension.purdue.edu/extmedia/ID/cafo/ID-350.pdf.

chicken wire. "We move the boxes every day to a fresh grassy spot so the land can regenerate."

"Is the grass irrigated?"

"No," she says. "It's rain-fed."

Until the Green Revolution, beginning in the 1950s, most agriculture was rain-fed. The Green Revolution (not to be confused with the Green Movement of present day) advocated irrigation technology to increase yields. During the next six decades, the use of pipes and sprinklers to bring water to fields tripled. Irrigation typically doubles yields, but it requires three times the amount of water.[113] The goal was to feed an exploding world population, with little concern for water conservation. In a water-scarce world, the challenge is to feed billions with less water.

We leave the chickens and walk toward the processing center, two plastic Rubbermaid tables in a clearing. Paul stands next to his step-daughter. He moves his hand over the skin of a plucked chicken to feel for bits of feathers.

"How do you dispose of the waste?" I ask Paul, noticing a small pile of chicken parts. He answers by walking me to the compost pile. I expect an odor like when you pass a CAFO on the highway and your nose flairs and crinkles in protest. I smell nothing but the nearby oranges hanging heavy on trees.

"This is several months' worth of discarded chicken parts and blood," says Paul. He stands next to the pile that comes up to his loosely tied ponytail. "After the pile is ready, we scatter the soil around the farm."

Chicken manure is absent from the mound of waste. The chickens directly fertilize the blades of grass they eat. This one-acre farm generates no gray water runoff, water tainted with nitrogen. The orchard absorbs the nutrient-rich compost.

---

113. Fred Pearce, *When the Rivers Run Dry: Water—The Defining Crisis of the Twenty-First Century* (Boston: Beacon Press, 2007): 11–12.

Conversely, chickens raised in CAFOs give rise to large amounts of gray water with the manure they leave behind. For example, a CAFO with 125,000 birds generates 9,375 pounds of manure every six weeks, the average lifetime of a broiler chicken.[114]

Customers begin to pull off the paved road onto the dirt. Darinka and Paul greet each customer like an old friend (some are). A scale sits on a table; fresh chickens float in coolers of ice and water.

"Why do you buy from Funny Farms?" I ask the first customer who arrives with her young daughter that Saturday afternoon. I want to know her motivation to drive beyond the edge of town and pay more than twice the price of a supermarket chicken.

"I know Darinka and Paul love their chickens. I see the way they care for them. Treating animals humanely is important to me," the woman answers. "And," she adds, "these are *great*-tasting chickens."

I drive home with my own fresh pasture-raised chicken I reserved in advance on the passenger seat. It will be ready for roasting after twenty-four hours.

---

114. Edward C. Naber and Alex J. Bermudez, "Poultry Manure Management and Utilization Problems and Opportunities," Bulletin 804, Ohio State University, 1990. Manure is between 70–80 percent moisture, accounting for the 75 percent loss of weight.

Funny Farm's Simple Roasted Chicken and Seasonal Vegetables

Makes 6 servings with leftovers

20 minutes to prepare

60 minutes to roast

In my kitchen, a whole chicken and roasted vegetables becomes two dinners and a handful of lunches. A favorite lunch is leftover roasted vegetables tossed with lettuce and some homemade vinaigrette dressing. Nothing is wasted. By stretching the chicken and vegetables over several meals, you reduce the water footprint of your food.

The tortilla soup recipe is inspired by the book *My Nepenthe*, named for a restaurant perched on the oceanside cliffs of Big Sur. With or without an ocean view, the soup is extraordinary.

I choose organic or pesticide-free, locally grown vegetables to minimize chemicals, heavy metals, and salt found in synthetic fertilizer runoff. Ask farmers whether they use rainwater or irrigation. If they use irrigation, ask if it is drip (the most water-efficient method) and support with your dollars those who implement water-sustainable practices.[115]

Ingredients

1 whole organic chicken that lived its life on grass, not concrete, aka pasture-raised, local (4–5 pounds), rinsed.

115. See "Chapter 3: Produce & Water."

3 teaspoons organic olive oil (dry farmed)[116]
3 teaspoons sea salt
½ teaspoon pepper
3 pounds seasonal organic vegetables, quartered
¼ cup chopped fresh rosemary or favorite herb from your garden

Directions

1. Preheat oven to 425°F.
2. In a large bowl, add seasonal vegetables, quartered. My favorites are beets, carrots, potatoes, red onions. Toss with 2 tablespoons of olive oil, 1½ teaspoons salt, ¼ teaspoon pepper and half the fresh rosemary. Mix with a spoon until all vegetables are coated. Pour vegetables into a 13×9-inch baking dish.
3. Prepare the chicken by placing it in the same bowl used for the vegetables to avoid wasting any leftover spices and oil. Rub the remaining spices and oil onto the exterior of the chicken. Nestle the chicken amongst the seasonal vegetables, breast side down.
4. Roast, spooning juices onto the vegetables and chicken occasionally, until a thermometer inserted into the thickest part of the chicken (avoid touching bone) registers 165°F, about 1 hour. (Start checking the chicken at 45 minutes.)
5. Before serving, let the chicken rest in a warm spot for 10 minutes. Serve with warm crusty bread.
6. Save your chicken bones, unused parts, and the carrot tops and pieces of unused onion. You can use these to make a simple chicken broth by boiling them in a pot of salted water. You can use the broth for the tortilla soup. If you won't be making stock immediately, put the uneaten chicken parts, bones, carrot and onion scraps in a bag and freeze.

---

116. See "Chapter 1: Wheat & Water."

Next-Night Chicken Tortilla Soup

Makes 6 servings

20 minutes to prepare

35 minutes to cook, additional 45 minutes if you make your own chicken broth from leftover chicken bones and parts

Ingredients

Leftover roasted chicken shredded into small-to-medium pieces (at least 1 cup)
2 tablespoons organic olive oil
6 organic tomatoes, diced
1 medium organic red onion, diced
1 organic jalapeño chile, seeded and minced (optional)
1 organic red bell pepper
8 cups homemade chicken broth (see step 6 in Roasted Chicken recipe)
2 organic limes
½ bunch organic fresh cilantro, stemmed and chopped
2 teaspoons ground cumin
2 teaspoons sea salt
1 teaspoon pepper
½ cup organic tomatillo salsa

GARNISHES

Organic tortilla chips

Shredded jack or cheddar cheese, preferably cheese from grazing cows[117]
Chopped fresh organic cilantro

Directions

1. Shred the chicken and set aside.
2. In a large pot, heat the oil. Add the tomatoes, onion, bell pepper, and chile and cook until soft, about 5 minutes.
3. Stir in the broth, lime juice, cilantro, cumin, salt, and pepper. Bring to a boil, then decrease the heat. Add the chicken and tomatillo salsa and cook for 20 minutes, or until all the flavors marry. Add additional salt, lime juice, and tomatillo salsa to suit your palette.
4. To serve, ladle the soup into bowls and top with tortilla chips, shredded cheese, and cilantro.

NOTE: To make your own tomatillo salsa, place 1 pound husked and rinsed tomatillos in a pot, cover with water and boil until soft. Roast 2 *chilies de arbol* on an iron skillet or *comal*, turning them a few times until they're charred on all sides. Discard the stems and some seeds. The more seeds you keep, the hotter the salsa. In a blender, combine tomatillos, 1 chopped onion, 2 cloves garlic, ½ bunch stemmed cilantro, and ⅓ cup water. Blend until smooth. Add more water for a thinner consistency. Season with salt and pepper to taste.

117. See "Chapter 9: Dairy & Water."

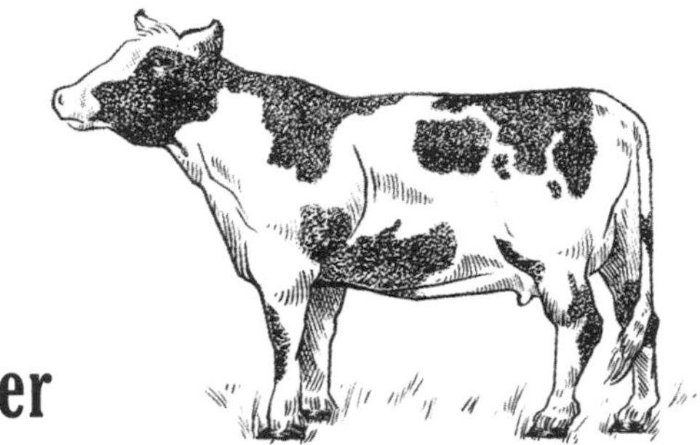

CHAPTER 9

Dairy & Water

1 glass of milk (8 ounces) = 45 gallons of water

1 pound of cheese = 414 gallons of water

1 gallon of milk = 720 gallons of water

1 pound of butter = 3,602 gallons of water[118]

"MEET THE GIRLS," says Paul Knapp, formally introducing me to the black-and-white spotted milk cows at Cobblestone Valley Farms. The cows impatiently wait indoors during the frigid winter for the verdant pastures of spring. In the meantime, Paul, dressed in mud-caked rubber boots and baseball cap, with help from his wife Maureen, shovels about fifty pounds of hay to the "girls," the average weight eaten by a dairy cow each day.[119]

Cobblestone Farms is among the 90 percent of rain-fed food acreage in the world. Rain-fed crops are grown with *green* water, diverting no water from the natural water cycle. In the last six decades, rain-fed pastures, like Cobblestone farms, have been in dramatic decline. Cows have been plucked off pastures and placed inside free stall barns constructed of steel or wood. Some of these buildings house upwards

118. Kostigen, *The Green Blue Book*.
119. "Dairy Facts," Purdue Food Animal Education Network, http://www.ansc.purdue.edu/faen/dairy%20facts.html.

of 3,000 cows.[120] These large dairies, classified by the USDA as Concentrated Animal Feeding Operations (CAFOs), are reliant on *blue* water—finite-resource groundwater and reservoirs—to irrigate crops of chemically treated corn, soy, and grain.[121]

"When do the cows return to the pasture?"

"Nature tells us when it's time. Some years it can be late April. Other years it's around the middle of May," Paul answers in his slow, steady tone.

"No matter what day it lands on, we and the cows are thankful," Maureen laughs. The grazing season is regional; the season for a cow in upstate New York may last six months. A cow in Northern California can graze all year. USDA organic certified dairy standards require cows to graze a minimum of four months of the grazing season.[122]

"Grazing was one of the first steps we took that led us to become organic," says Paul as we walk a short distance to the field. Faint green grass is peppered over the 300 acres.

"When we first learned how to graze cattle, we would put the cows out after every milking on a new pasture, which kept the grass short, about six to eight inches long. The problem is short grass is high in protein. Dairy cows need protein to grow and produce milk, but short grass has too much protein, especially in the spring," says Maureen. "What

---

120. James M. MacDonald et al., "Profits, Costs, and the Changing Structure of Dairy Farming," USDA, September 2007, http://usda.proworks.com/publications/pub-details/?pubid=112972. The EPA defines a large dairy CAFO as having more than 700 mature cattle.

121. "Profiling Food Consumption in America," *Agricultural Fact Book*, USDA: 13–21, https://assets.documentcloud.org/documents/2461300/usda-chapter2.pdf. The water footprint of dairy is 48,971 gallons. To calculate this total I used the USDA totals of dairy consumption for each dairy product (2,000). I referred to *The Green Blue Book* for water footprint totals for each category. A specific total was unavailable for frozen dairy products (ice cream, frozen yogurt, sherbet); therefore I assumed the water footprint to be the same as for cream.

122. "USDA Issues Final Rule on Organic Access to Pasture," USDA AMS, December 2010, https://www.ams.usda.gov/press-release/usda-issues-final-rule-organic-access-pasture. The new USDA requirement replaces the "access to pasture" rule, which invited a multitude of definitions by the industry.

we learned is if you let the grass grow taller, it gives the cows more choice. They can eat a balance of protein-rich grass lower to the ground and taller energy-giving grass."

"The cows intuitively know if they need tall grass or short grass?"

"Yes, that's exactly it. The method is called holistic management."

Holistic management, also called planned or mob grazing, mimics nature by corralling animals on a small piece of pasture and moving them to a fresh spot before the patch is overgrazed. This farm technique is based on the findings of South African biologist Allan Savory. In the African grasslands, he observed how large herds of herbivores moved across the plain and grazed one area. The uneaten pasture mixed with their excrement was ground into the soil by their hoofs. The threat of predators kept the herds moving before an area was overgrazed. This process increased the vitality of the soil. The herds returned to the same pasture the following season to find it grown back.[123]

"Before we used holistic management, the grass dried out in the summer, and we supplemented the cows' diet with soybeans. Now the cows rely on the pasture with a small amount of grain mixture," says Maureen.

"Why?"

"We move them off the pasture quicker, leaving more of the vegetative cover on the ground. The vegetative cover shades the ground and allows seeds to germinate and fill in bare spots. The roots from the grass feed the microbes in the soil and build the organic matter that retains more water. More water held in the ground is good for the pasture and good for the adjoining river," says Maureen.

The Savory Institute found organic matter to increase by 2–3 percent on holistic-managed land after three to five years. For each 1 percent

---

123. Tony Malmberg (co-founder of the Savory Institute and a practitioner of holistic management) in discussion with the author, March 2013. Allen Savory, "How to fight desertification and reverse climate change," TED, February 2013, https://www.ted.com/talks/allan_savory_how_to_green_the_world_s_deserts_and_reverse_climate_change.

increase of organic soil, water retention increases by 20,000 to 25,000 gallons per acre, equivalent to enough water to fill 804 bathtubs.[124]

~

Paul and Maureen lead me to the last unexplored building across from the barn. Inside, two dozen cows linger along the perimeters of the milking room. "This is a lot of cows to milk."

"Not really. There are herds in California with easily 500 cows," Maureen continues. "We have about eighty dairy cows and about the same number of younger calves to take their place." The majority of organic dairy farms are small. In fact, 87 percent of organic dairy farms in the United States have fewer than one hundred cows.[125]

"The cows are milked with a vacuum system placed on the udder, and the milk moves from the hoses into the pipes and is pumped into the tank," says Paul, pointing at the stainless steal pipes hanging from the rafters in straight lines and right angles.

"Do you want to see the milk?" Maureen asks. I nod. They lead me to the adjoining room simply called the "milk room." Inside, Paul lifts the lid of a round steel tank that occupies most of the small space.

"Here's two days' worth."

I peer into the tank. The white milk is bright against the steel gray. "It looks beautiful," Maureen and Paul laugh with pride.

---

124. Dave Mengel, "Agronomy E-Updates," Kansas State University K-State Research and Extension, https://webapp.agron.ksu.edu/agr_social/eu.throck; K.T. Weber and B.S. Gokhale, "Effect Of Grazing On Soil-Water Content in Semiarid Rangelands of Southeast Idaho," *Journal of Arid Environments* 75 (2011): 464–70. I used the average of 22,250 gallons per acre and multiplied with the average SOM increase of holistic management lands of 2.5 percent. I divided this total of 56,250 gallons per acre with 70 gallons, the average of water used in a bath.

125. William D. McBride and Catherine Greene, "Characteristics, Costs, and Issues for Organic Dairy Farming," USDA Economic Research Service, November 2009. More than 80 percent of US organic dairies are located in the Northeast and Midwest. The West has fewer organic dairies but has larger herds averaging 381 cows. The West accounts for one-third of all organic milk totals.

The loud rumble of a diesel engine pours into the milk house. The Organic Valley Family of Farms semi-truck arrives to siphon the creamy white milk. Cobblestone Valley Farms is a member of the Organic Valley cooperative.

"Where will this milk go?"

Maureen yells over the diesel engine, "We're a national co-op, but we do things on a regional basis. For the most part, the milk stays local. Each region collects, packages, and redistributes the milk to local outlets."

We walk back to the barn. "As conventional farmers, we knew nothing about the milk once it left the farm," says Paul.

Paul's great-grandfather began the dairy farm over one hundred years earlier. It began as a small pasture-based operation, but evolved over the decades along with the US dairy industry. The cows were fed grain instead of grass, the herd grew, and growth hormones and antibiotics applied to the feed increased milk production. After acquiring the dairy, Paul and Maureen gradually returned the farm to a small, pasture-based operation and began the conversion to organic in 1998.

"Do your cows produce less milk or more milk now that you've converted to an organic pasture-centered dairy?"

"Milk production has gone down. Grain-fed cows produce more milk," answers Maureen.

"What does it mean for your bottom line?"

"We don't produce as much milk, but we make more money because feeding cows grain is expensive," she says.

While organic dairies are found to produce 30 percent less, milk production on conventional dairy farms increased by 32 percent since the introduction of growth hormones in 1994.[126] The modern cow pro-

126 . I compared 1993, the year before FDA approval of the rBST on dairy farms, with 2012, the latest milk USDA production statistics. The exact milk pounds per cow are: 15,722 (1993); 21,697 (2012). Data found through the USDA National Agricultural Statistics Service (NASS) here: http://usda.mannlib.cornell.edu/MannUsda/viewDocumentInfo.do?documentID=1103.

duces almost four times more milk than a cow in the year 1950.[127] The increase in milk is explained by the mechanization of farm operation, the shift in diet, and the use of synthetic hormones. Growth hormones like rBST (also referred to as rBGH) developed by US-based chemical company Monsanto Corporation can boost production by 10–20 percent per cow.[128]

Of all the hormones discharged by livestock in the United States, 90 percent originate from dairy farms.[129] According to a study published in the *Journal of Environmental Science and Technology*, concentrations of hormones in agricultural waste are 100–1,000 times higher than in human sewage. Hormone-tainted water is linked to the *feminization* of fish, also called *gender-bending*. Gender-bending is the development of egg cells in testes or the growth of female reproductive ducts in male fish.[130] Although some fish species are known to switch genders naturally, the rate of occurrences is unnatural. Gender-bending a fish hinders its ability to reproduce, placing further downward pressure on already stressed fish populations.[131]

Over a nine-year period, scientists from the US Geological Survey found gender-bending in every lake, stream, and river tested. One ex-

---

127. James M. MacDonald et al., "Profits, Costs, and the Changing Structure of Dairy Farming," USDA, September 2007, http://usda.proworks.com/publications/pub-details/?pubid=112972. According to USDA Agricultural statistics, a cow produced 5,314 pounds of milk in 1950 and 18,204 in 2000.

128. "Dairy," Sustainable Table, http://gracelinks.org/media/pdf/dairy_tp_20090515.pdf. W. D. Dobson, "The BST case" in *Government and the Food Industry: Economic and Political Effects of Conflict and Co-Operation*, L. Tim Wallace and William R. Schroder, eds., (Springer, 1997):141–158.

129. Wei Zheng et al., "Anaerobic Transformation Kinetics and Mechanism of Steroid Estrogenic Hormones in Dairy Lagoon Water," *Environmental Science & Technology* 46 (2012): 5471–478.

130. Karen L. Thorpe et al., "Relative Potencies and Combination Effects of Steroidal Estrogens in Fish," *Environmental Science & Technology* 37, no. 6, (2003): 1142–149.

131. Christopher Joyce, "Study: Gender-Bending Fish Widespread In US," NPR, September 16, 2009, http://www.npr.org/templates/story/story.php?storyId=112888785. Scientist with the US Geological Services found 18 percent of largemouth bass and 33 percent of smallmouth bass to have intersex.

ception was Alaska's Yukon River. Alaska is home to only five dairies statewide.[132]

"The use of rBST results in more milk initially, but after one or two lactations the cow is auctioned for ground beef. A cow produces milk after her first calf and is impregnated once each year to maintain her milk. A lactation cycle refers to each time a cow gives birth."

"What is the average number of lactation cycles for your herd?"

"Our average is six to seven lactations. We have cows that produce for ten, eleven, twelve lactations," Maureen says.

"Three times more lactation cycles!" The disparity surprises me. "Why would hormones shorten the lifespan so dramatically?"

"What happens to the cow can be compared to an engine running at full capacity," Maureen continues. "It starts strong, but soon parts of the engine begin to break down. Something similar occurs to a cow on rBST. She is producing an unnatural amount of milk; her biological processes are disrupted, and pretty soon body systems begin to break down. Mastitis, inflammation of the mammary gland, is usually the first symptom. The response is antibiotics, which further disrupt the cow's systems, and on it goes; the result being irreparable damage, so the cow is sold as meat."

"Slowly farmers are beginning to realize this practice is unsustainable," adds Paul. "They're losing money in the deal because hormones don't increase milk in the long term of a cow's lifetime on a conventional farm versus a farm like ours."

Nationwide, growth hormone use has fallen from 18 percent in 2000 to 9 percent in 2012.[133] Small farms tend to use the growth hormone the most sparingly, with use at 2 percent. But as the herd sizes

---

132. Ellen Lockyear, "Is Alaska's Dairy Industry Making a Comeback? Or on the Brink?," *Progressive Dairyman Magazine*, June 7, 2011, http://www.progressivedairy.com/news/industry-news/is-alaskas-dairy-industry-making-a-comeback-or-on-the-brink.

133. "Milk Production Costs and Returns per Hundredweight Sold, By Size Group," USDA Economic Research Service, 2012, https://www.ers.usda.gov/data-products/milk-cost-of-production-estimates.aspx.

increase so does the usage of growth hormones. Growth hormones are dispensed to 22 percent of dairy cows in herds of 500–999.[134]

The USDA organic rules ban synthetic hormones on all certified organic livestock.[135] Fewer than 3 percent of US dairy cows are organic certified, accounting for less than 3 percent of all milk sold.[136]

~

My attention is caught by mason jars tucked in the woodwork of the barn. Each is filled with small white tablets. "What's inside the jars?"

"We uses homeopathy in lieu of antibiotics." Paul looks over at Maureen and smiles at her while he explains. "Maureen has studied homeopathy extensively and uses it for the animals and the family." I look at both of them, together in the milk room, silently recognizing their partnership.

"Is the use of homeopathy a standard practice for organic dairy farms?"

---

134. Ibid. The smallest farms are defined as less than fifty milk cows.
135. To curb antibiotic resistance in humans caused by growth hormone used on livestock, the Food and Drug Administration (FDA) in late 2013 asked for "voluntary cooperation" from the drug industry to remove drugs similar to drugs administered on humans to be removed from growth promoters. For more on human antibiotic resistance see "Chapter 10: Meat & Water." USDA organic rules state that if the animal is ill, there is an approved list of synthetic drugs. For the complete list of requirements, see https://www.ams.usda.gov/sites/default/files/media/Organic%20Livestock%20Requirements.pdf.
136. "Certified Organic Livestock, 2011, by State," USDA Economic Research Service, 2011, https://www.ers.usda.gov/data-products/organic-production. The total number of organic dairy cows was 254,771 in 2011. The largest number of certified organic milk cows resided in California (57,809) followed by Wisconsin (31,874) and New York (28,446). The totals do not include young stock. The total number of milk cows in the US during the same period was 9,233,000. "Milk Production Costs and Returns per Hundredweight Sold, 2011–2012," USDA Economic Research Service, https://www.ers.usda.gov/data-products/milk-cost-of-production-estimates.aspx. 2.77 percent of all milk sold in the United States was USDA certified organic in both 2011 and 2012.

"Not all, but many do use homeopathy for their animals," says Maureen. The use of antibiotics is common on conventional dairies as both prevention and treatment, but prohibited on USDA certified organic dairies. According to a study published in the *Journal of Antimicrobial Chemotherapy*, US farms dispensed 16,000 tons of antibiotics for livestock in 2008 alone, eight times more than the antibiotics used to treat humans.[137] Regulations require the milk of a lactating cow treated with antibiotics to be disposed of, but there are no additional regulations for the treatment of waste.[138]

"I've never realized how often cows relieve themselves," I watch manure tumble to the ground from the animals near me.

"They keep on giving," says Paul. We all laugh.

The amount of waste accumulating in dairies around the country is no laughing matter. The amount of waste swells with larger herd sizes. The waste from the estimated 450,000 dairy cows in Tulare County, California, alone, the producer of the most milk of any county in the United States, is five times more than the sewage from the New York City metro area.[139]

The standard waste management practice is to store the raw manure anywhere from several days to several months and transport it to nearby crop fields to be used as fertilizer. With raw manure, the nitrogen is readily available to the plants. But often there is not enough cropland to receive the tremendous levels of nitrogen in such quantities of raw manure. The excess nitrogen from the raw manure unused by the plant is lost to air and water.

---

137. K. Kummerer, "Significance of Antibiotics in the Environment," *Journal of Antimicrobial Chemotherapy* 52 (2003): 5–7, http://jac.oxfordjournals.org/content/52/1/5.full.
138. Nicole Neeser, DVM, "Antibiotic Use in Production Agriculture," University of Minnesota College of Veterinary Medicine, May 2003, http://www.poultryu.umn.edu/publications-resources/antibiotic-use.
139. "Factory Farm Map," Food and Water Watch, http://www.factoryfarmmap.org.

In the air, the nitrogen converts to ammonia, a contributor to climate change. Of all the ammonia GHG emissions in the United States, 50–70 percent is emitted from an animal operation. In water, the excess nutrients are lost as nitrates, the soluble form of nitrogen.[140] A report by the USDA calculates 95 percent of nitrogen ingested by an animal is excreted in its waste, a major contaminant of rivers and lakes.[141]

"Where does the manure go? Do you have to shovel it out?"

Maureen laughs at my question.

"There's a chain with paddles," she says. "It's like a conveyor belt that carries the manure up into the chute and out onto a spreader." We follow the conveyor belt outside. She points to a square cement structure nearby. "That's the manure storage. Some manure we spread on our fields and the rest becomes compost."

In compost, the nitrogen and other nutrients beneficial to the plant release slowly. In this way, the leaching of nitrogen into the water and air is drastically minimized. Compost with high levels of organic matter increases the ability of the soil to hold moisture. Combined, composting and grazing contribute to cleaner air and water while providing nutrients to the grasses and the farm's pick-your-own strawberry fields open in the summer months.

"See those long, narrow mounds? Those are windrows." Paul points in the direction of the pasture. The compost hills are shallow, about knee-height, and extend for several yards.

"Do you have any lining underneath?"

---

140. Claudia Copeland, "Animal Waste and Water Quality: EPA's Response to the Waterkeeper Alliance Court Decision on Regulation of CAFOs," Rep. no. 7-5700, Congressional Research Service, 2011; Marcel Aillery et al., "Chapter 2: Animal Agriculture and the Environment," *Managing Manure to Improve Air and Water Quality* (Washington, DC: USDA, Economic Research Service, 2005).

141. Ibid. The fish most affected by large fish kills resulting from manure spills include minnows, gar, largemouth bass, striped bass, and flounder.

"We use compost pads underneath, but runoff isn't a concern. The carbon from the plant material collects the nitrogen, absorbing the nutrients," says Paul.

"The recipe for compost is nitrogen and carbon?"

"Exactly," he answers, "but we need much more carbon than nitrogen to make good compost. We use the bedding from the stalls for the carbon, but it's not enough. We partner with our local municipality for their wood chips, leaves, and other green waste."

Maureen adds, "The downside to using municipal waste is the trash. I don't think people realize the trash they throw in their green waste bins isn't sorted out. The garbage gets shredded with the green waste, mixed with the compost, and scattered on cropland or pastures. I think if households knew this, we would see less trash."

A creek slices through the pasture. Along the creek, naked maple trees wait expectantly for spring. The tributary that leads to the Tioughnioga River led the Knapps to convert their dairy operation from conventional to organic fifteen years earlier.

"For many years we never gave much thought to what went into the water," says Paul.

"We never considered the runoff. We would take the cows to the water to drink and drive them through the river to graze on the field on the other side."

"What made you think about the river?"

"The epiphany came when we started to work with the Soil and Water Conservation District. They told us we are at the headwaters of the Chesapeake watershed. The water from this tributary dumps into the Bay." Paul walks us toward the stream.

One hundred fifty rivers and streams spanning six states spill their water into Chesapeake Bay, making it the largest estuary in the United States and one of the largest in the world. The inlet's brackish water teems with life and is home to 300 species of birds and fish.

The Chesapeake Bay is home to a 'dead zone,' the first oxygen-deprived water discovered in the United States. The dead zone grows in the underwater of the Bay, fed by pollutants upstream. Discharge of nutrients from agriculture is responsible for at least 50 percent of the pollution.[142] Fish, crabs, and shellfish struggle to survive in the murky water. Oysters called "Chesapeake white gold" for their treasured flavor perish with other shellfish.[143]

Former President Obama issued an Executive Order in 2009 to declare the Bay a "national treasure." He called on the federal government to "lead the effort" to restore the estuary.[144] The EPA, in collaboration with other federal agencies, issued a strategy to protect the Chesapeake with stricter rules than the revised Clean Water Act (CWA) of 2008.[145] It includes rules on storm water and pollution discharges from animal feedlots (currently storm water run-off from agricultural operations is exempt under the CWA).[146]

---

142. Darryl Fears, "Alarming 'Dead Zone' Grows in the Chesapeake," *Washington Post,* July 24, 2011, https://www.washingtonpost.com/national/health-science/alarming-dead-zone-grows-in-the-chesapeake/2011/07/20/gIQABRmKXI_story.html?utm_term=.de2404e56e45; Claudia Copeland, "Animal Waste and Water Quality."

143. Kendra B. Morris, "Consider the Chesapeake Bay Oyster," *Kitchen Window,* NPR, November 21, 2007, http://www.npr.org/templates/story/story.php?storyId=16369187.

144. "Executive Order 13508—Chesapeake Bay Protection and Restoration," The White House, May 12, 2009, http://web.archive.org/web/20170117150755/https://www.whitehouse.gov/the-press-office/executive-order-chesapeake-bay-protection-and-restoration. For updated information regarding information on the executive order and progress toward restoring the Chesapeake Bay visit http://executiveorder.chesapeakebay.net.

145. Marcel Aillery et al., "Chapter 2: Animal Agriculture and the Environment," "Managing Manure to Improve Air and Water Quality," USDA Economic Research Service, September 2005: 3–11, https://www.ers.usda.gov/webdocs/publications/46336/28992_err9fm.pdf?v=41102. The Clean Water Act, established in 1972, protects "all permanent, standing or continuously flowing bodies of water." These include oceans, rivers, lakes, streams, etc. Groundwater is protected by the Safe Drinking Water Act, Resource Conservation and Recovery Act, and the Superfund Act. Private wells are not covered.

146. Claudia Copeland, "Animal Waste and Water Quality."

The Clean Water Act (CWA), signed into law by Former President Nixon in 1972, is responsible for the regulation of pollutant discharges into the nation's waters. The nation's waters include oceans, rivers, lakes, streams, but don't include groundwater or private wells.

In 2003, the CWA revised its rules to address the growing frequency of major fish kills resulting from manure waste spills from CAFOs. The revised rules are intended to reduce the amount of nutrients, mainly nitrogen, introduced into surface-water resources. The most controversial of the new rules was the "duty to apply" requirement, mandating all CAFOs apply for an EPA-issued permit requiring waste discharges to be monitored and reported. A federal court decision, resulting from legal challenges, vacated this rule. Under the *watered-down* revised rules, CAFOs can *voluntarily* seek permits.

"What we do affects people from here to the Chesapeake," says Paul. "The more we thought about it, the more we felt we never want to be in a position that causes a negative effect downstream. It is the biggest reason we became an organic dairy."

"We also sit above a large aquifer. It goes all along the valley and is the main source of water for the area," adds Maureen.

"When you think about it, we all live upstream." On those words, Paul walks toward the weathered white barn, to the "girls" awaiting his shovels of hay.

Maureen drives me back to my car parked near her denim-blue, two-story house built by Paul's great-grandfather. Maureen has one last thing to share with me. A field broadcaster is tucked away behind a shed near the house like a secret. It is no more than a white PVC pipe jutting upwards from the ground.

Maureen learned about field broadcasters in her research on biodynamic farming.[147] It is believed the positive intentions placed inside

147. See "Chapter 13: Wine & Water" to learn about biodynamic farming.

the field broadcaster resonate over the surrounding area. Maureen borrowed the idea for their organic farm.

Stuffed inside the pipe is a map of the farm and a letter she wrote.

"Will you read your letter to me?" I ask.

"Sure," her voice becomes quiet. She had never read her letter to anyone outside her family. She stands in front of her field broadcaster. The sound of the interstate highway roaring behind us forces her to raise her voice:

> *We give our love freely to our farm and beyond. We shower the soil, plant life, water, air with our thoughts of great bounty. We welcome the energy from the stars, planets, and the universe. We work every day with love and gratitude in our heart . . . We learn, build, and maintain a healthy environment. We look forward to abundant and nutritious production of the highest quality food possible for the benefit of all . . .*

The dairy farm operations hold the rhythm of her words, as does the milk that left the farm now traveling on I-81 in an Organic Valley truck.

Cobblestone Farm's Crustless Cheesecake with Fresh Strawberry Topping

Makes 12 servings

30 minutes to prepare

60 minutes to bake, additional 60 minutes with oven off

20 minutes to cook optional fruit topping

This recipe is as easy as it is creamy. Don't let the "preparing for the bath" instruction or the requirement of a 9-inch springform pan discourage you. If you're a novice baker like me, you will need to buy a springform pan. Trust me, the small investment is worth its weight in sweet, cheesy decadence that seeps into the pores of your tongue like spring rain on healthy soil.

Ingredients

2 pounds Organic Valley cream cheese
1¼ cups fair-trade organic sugar
4 large organic pasture-raised eggs
2 teaspoons organic vanilla extract
¼ cup Organic Valley heavy cream
¼ cup Organic Valley sour cream

Directions

1. Preheat oven to 325°F.
2. Separate the bottom of the 9-inch springform pan from the ring. Line the bottom with foil. Tuck the excess foil underneath (be sure the foil is large enough to cover the sides of pan). Place the foil-lined bottom back inside the ring and clamp in place. Pull the excess foil from the underside of the pan up around the side of the pan.
3. To prepare for a bath, cover the outside of the pan (bottom and ring) with heavy-duty foil. Set the springform pan inside a roasting pan. Boil water in a separate pan or kettle to be used for the bath.
4. Beat cream cheese in a bowl until smooth. Add sugar gradually and beat until dissolved.
5. Add 1 egg at a time and incorporate into the batter. After each egg, scrape down the cream cheese that sticks to the sides of the bowl. Add the vanilla.
6. Stir in the heavy cream and sour cream.
7. Pour the batter into prepared springform pan and nest inside the roasting pan. Pour boiling water inside the roasting pan until it comes halfway up the outside of the springform pan. Place the roasting pan inside the oven.
8. Bake for 55–60 minutes. The cake will jiggle in the center, but the perimeter should be baked. To bake the center without cracking the cheesecake, turn off the oven but leave the door ajar and let the cake bake for an additional hour.
9. Remove the submerged springform pan from the roasting pan and place on a wire rack to cool. Once it's at room temperature, cover and refrigerate for about 4 hours. Serve plain, or for more sweet decadence, add fruit topping. See the recipe below.

Fruit Topping Ingredients

1 cup fresh organic strawberries (you can substitute any berries)

⅓–½ cup fair-trade sugar (sweeten to taste)

1 tablespoon arrowroot or cornstarch

Fruit Topping Directions

1. Crush half of the berries in a small saucepan. Add sugar and let juice form, about 20 minutes.
2. Add the remaining whole berries and cook over medium heat until thick and clear, stirring often.
3. Add warm fruit topping after the cheesecake has been refrigerated.
4. Pour over the cake from the center; it will pool out to the edges. Refrigerate till firm.

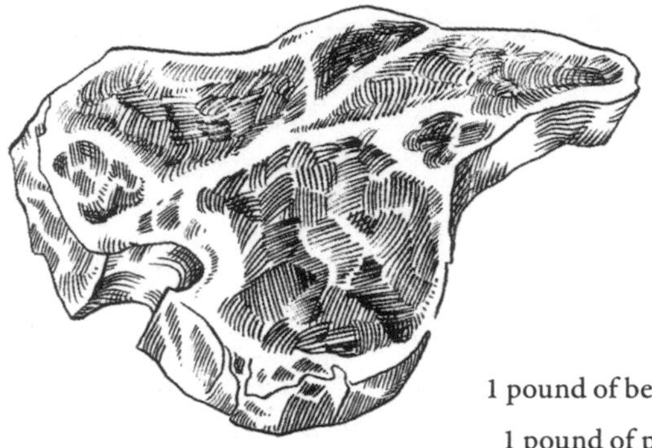

CHAPTER 10
Meat & Water

1 pound of beef = 1,851 gallons of water[148]
1 pound of pork = 631 gallons of water[149]
1 pound of lamb = 398.8 gallons of water[150]

LIVESTOCK IS THE largest user and polluter of water. The search for the *best* raised meat for water and the environment led me to Hunter Cattle near Savannah, Georgia. Their livestock will not step one hoof in a feedlot, where grain and corn replace pasture and the accumulation of their excrement waste would leech into water systems. Nor are the cows allowed to graze continuously on a wide open pasture, trample on sensitive ecosystems, or pollute streams and rivers. Instead, the animals rotate onto fenced-off paddocks every few days. Sheep follow the cows, eating the plants and weeds the cattle leave behind. Pasture is never irrigated, or treated with chemicals, both leading causes of water scarcity. Manure is absorbed by the land, building organic matter in the soil (SOM) which absorbs water. In this system, the land is not overgrazed.

---

148. Arjen Y. Hoekstra, "The hidden water resource use behind meat and dairy," *Animal Frontiers* 2, no. 2 (April 2012): 3–8, http://waterfootprint.org/media/downloads/Hoekstra-2012-Water-Meat-Dairy.pdf.
149. Thomas Kostigen, *The Green Blue Book: The Simple Water-Savings Guide to Everything in Your Life* (Emmaus, PA: Rodale, 2010). The water footprint of cured meat is higher at 676.3 gallons.
150. Ibid.

The *managed intensive grazing* systems implemented at Hunter Cattle are among the *best* examples of animal operations. Hunter's system works to reverse decades of soil erosion, pollution, GHG emissions, dead zones, and lowered ground water levels—modern-day environmental disasters all traced back to livestock.

~

"*He's* driving us?" I ask Kristan Fretwell, co-owner of Hunter Cattle along with her extended family. She slides in next to her ten-year-old son Forrest already seated behind the wheel.[151]

"Shoot, he's a better driver than me," she says of her eldest child. Whether it is her sweet tea–soaked Georgia accent or her big, easy smile, I believe her. I take my spot in the passenger seat. Forrest revs the engine of the Pioneer, an all-terrain vehicle, and drives toward the pasture.

"We leave the woods intact," says Kristen, pointing to a thick grove of trees. "These acres are pasture, but much of the 300 acres is wooded. We think it is super important for the animals to have the shelter of the woods."

Forrest shuts off the engine, letting us off at a wooded area next to a paddock.

The world's forests sequester 8.8 billion tons of carbon dioxide.[152] But the world's forests are vanishing. The United Nations estimates eighteen million acres are deforested annually, mostly for cattle raising. In Brazil alone, the global leader in beef exports, cattle are responsible for

151. Kristen Fretwell and Forrest Fretwell in discussion with the author, July 2016.
152. Mark Clayton, "Study: Forests absorb much more greenhouse gas than previously known," *Christian Science Monitor*, July 15, 2011, http://www.csmonitor.com/Environment/2011/0715/Study-Forests-absorb-much-more-greenhouse-gas-than-previously-known.

75 percent of the deforestation in the Amazon. Eighty million cows overgraze pasture carved from the most biodiverse rainforest in the world.[153]

Standing next to the pasture, Kristan says, "Take a deep breath."

I do as she instructs.

"What do you smell?"

"Fresh air, grass, bark," I say.

"I ask everyone I bring here if they smell anything bad."

"Toxic waste runoff is one of the biggest issues for feedlots or overgrazed pasture," she says. "There ain't nothing toxic about this poop; it's grass and hay. Our manure doesn't run off anywhere. It's all absorbed by the soil. People ask us often if we will sell them our manure, but we don't have any extra to sell. It's composted into the land, building our soil. And the animals are not allowed in rivers or streams, keeping their waste out of the water. Nitrates or bacteria have never been found in our well or river. The well water is tested every month. Our water is so good and nutritious that our employees bring bottles to fill and take home."

For land to benefit from the nutrient-rich excrement of livestock, the number of animals cannot exceed the capacity of the receiving land to absorb the nutrients. The EPA reports nutrient pollution as the leading cause of "water quality impairment" in lakes and estuaries; second in rivers, behind sediment.[154] Concentrated animal feeding operations (CAFO), defined as animal feeding operations (AFO) with greater than 1,000 animals, generate extraordinary amounts of waste. As of January 1, 2016, there were ninety-two million cattle and calves excreting nutrients in the United States, approximately one cow for every three Americans.[155]

153. Rhett A. Butler, "Brazilian beef giant announces moratorium on rainforest beef," *Conservation News*, August 13, 2009, https://news.mongabay.com/2009/08/brazilian-beef-giant-announces-moratorium-on-rainforest-beef.

154. Nitrogen, the more soluble of both nutrients, is effortlessly transported into water systems by runoff, leachate, and tile drainage, the term used to describe the removal of excess water on subsoil.

155. "Beef Industry Statistics," National Cattlemen's Beef Association, http://www.beefusa.org/beefindustrystatistics.aspx.

I look down and see I'm standing on dried cow poop. It crumples underneath my sandal. The pasture is scattered with manure in different stages of decomposition. The advantage to a pasture-based animal operation is the natural spread of nitrogen rich manure on the land.

For CAFOs with no crops, transporting manure to nearby farms offers a partial fix. A USDA study found the cost of hauling manure from large feedlots (more than 500 cattle) to exceed its nutrient value beyond a nine-mile radius. But most counties don't have enough local cropland to absorb the abundance of manure generated.[156] The University of Minnesota calculates 50 percent of nitrogen in manure turns to vapor or gas before it's moved to cropland.[157] States with high concentrations of CAFOs experience on average twenty to thirty serious water quality problems per year caused by the overabundance of animal excrement. In an inventory conducted by the EPA, twenty-nine states identified AFOs and CAFOs as contributing to "water quality impairment," water too dirty to drink.[158]

Drawn by our voices, the cows move closer to the fence. Together they sound like whining cats. "Cows are curious, like gossiping women," she says. I laugh at the comparison.

"How many paddocks do you have?" I ask.

"We have eight or nine fields. To be honest with you, we would like these pastures to be cut in half because they don't need to be so big. It's better for the land when the animals are closer together. We can raise

156. B. Eghball and J.F. Power, "Management of Manure From Beef Cattle in Feedlots and From Minor Classes of Livestock," USDA Agricultural Research Services, 1994: 45–59, https://www.ars.usda.gov/is/np/agbyproducts/agbychap2.pdf.
157. C. M. Zehnder and A. DiCostanzo, "Estimating Feedlot Nutrient Budgets and Managing Manure Output," University of Minnesota Department of Animal Science, 2012, http://www.extension.umn.edu/agriculture/beef/components/nutmgmt.htm.
158. Carrie Hribar, MA, "Understanding Concentrated Animal Feeding Operations and Their Impact on Communities," Center for Disease Control National Association of Local Boards of Health, 2010, https://www.cdc.gov/nceh/ehs/docs/understanding_cafos_nalboh.pdf.

cows on a lot less land. We raise one cow on one acre versus the average of two to five acres of land."

"Will smaller paddocks affect the rotation?"

"Yes, the smaller the paddock, the faster the animals are moved off the land to keep it from being overgrazed," says Kristan.

Most cattle around the world spend the early part of their life on pasture, and the final three to six months being fattened up on a feedlot.[159] While open pastures are superior to feedlots in regards to health and the environment, they are land-intensive and give rise to overgrazing, the leading cause of desertification.[160]

The cows at Hunter Cattle return to a paddock after the land has regenerated: this is the main distinction among grass-fed cows in continuous-grazed vs. managed-grazed systems. Managed-grazed land like at Hunter Cattle builds carbon in the soil. Carbon-rich soils are beneficial. Carbon, the leading greenhouse gas (GHG), when kept in the ground increases the holding ability of water, and defends the land against droughts and severe rain events. Overgrazed land releases the GHG. In the last 200 years, the soil in the US has lost over half of its carbon.[161]

~

The cows' mooing crescendos. "They're talking to the cows on the other field," Kristan says.

"What do you mean?"

---

159. William D. McBride and Kenneth Mathews, "The Diverse Structure and Organization of US Beef Cow-Calf Farms," USDA Economic Research Service, March 2011, https://www.ers.usda.gov/topics/farm-economy/farm-structure-and-organization/research-on-farm-structure-and-organization.aspx.
160. Allen Savory, "How to fight desertification and reverse climate change," TED, February 2013, https://www.ted.com/talks/allan_savory_how_to_green_the_world_s_deserts_and_reverse_climate_change.
161. See "Chapter 6: Soy, Corn & Water."

"You know the expression 'the grass is always greener on the other side'? The cows are always excited to get elsewhere."

"I suppose humans aren't that different from cows."

"That's exactly right. You don't even need to herd the cows to another pasture. We call them, open the fence, and they walk through the gate to get to the grass on the other side."

White egrets stand motionless on the pasture. Kristan calls them cowbirds. "These birds got the cows' backs literally. They sit on their backs and eat all the bugs off them. The other day a cow had three birds on it. That was one lucky cow."

"How do you treat your cows when they get sick?" I ask.

"They don't get sick. The worst they get is pink eye."

"Really, your animals never get sick?"

"No. Why would they? They are out in nature, eating exactly what they were intended to eat," she says.

Overall, 80 percent of all antibiotics used in the United States are administered to livestock. Feed of grain and corn, engineered for maximum weight gain on a feedlot, disrupts the natural process of ruminant digestion. This unnatural diet leads to numerous maladies for a cow; chief among them are abscesses in the liver.[162] Antibiotics added to feed and water help to prevent such illnesses and keep the cow growing at a fast pace. The widespread use of non-therapeutic antibiotics in cattle feed poses a complex set of challenges, including the emergence of dangerous Shiga toxin–producing E. coli (STEC) strains.[163]

E. coli bacteria live in the intestines of animals and humans alike and contribute to a healthy intestinal tract. Overexposure to antibiotics over time, however, has evolved robust strains of STEC bacteria, with

---

162. James B. Russell, *Rumen microbiology and its role in ruminant nutrition* (Ithaca, NY: Dept. of Microbiology, Cornell University, 2002).

163. Non-therapeutic antibiotic use refers to administering antibiotics when the animal is not sick. Therapeutic use refers to the use of antibiotics exclusively when an animal is sick for a defined period.

E. coli 0157 being the most well-known.[164] According to the Center for Disease Control (CDC), 265,000 STEC infections in humans occur each year in the US alone. The greatest source of human exposure to these strains, according to the CDC, is from cattle manure scattered on cropland.

"When we started twelve years ago there were no fences. No planted fields," says Kristan. "All we knew was we wanted grass-fed cows because that's what they're designed to eat."

A cow is a ruminant animal. Deer, elk, buffalo, sheep, giraffes, and camels also belong to this club of grass eaters. These animals have four stomachs designed to process vegetation. Through a system of fermentation, the ruminant stomach, (the rumen, the largest among the four), extracts nutrients for the animal and passes along excrement, ripe with microorganisms ready to build the soil.[165]

"When we started, we didn't know anything about farming. The first steak from one of our cows, we chewed, sucked all the nutrition out, and spat it out." She laughs. "But this is how the Lord works, because we ended up meeting a neighbor who's a farmer and meat scientist. He said, 'Y'all there is so much more to raising grass-fed cows than just putting them on any kind of grass. There's a science behind it.' That's when we started planting different types of grasses."

In the summer, the family plants four different native grasses; in the winter, rye and clover. Seeds are planted directly into the decomposing plant material from the previous season in a no-till system. Tillage overturns the soil, and is the favored method for cropland across the nation. But the unearthing of the soil by tillers releases carbon into the atmosphere.[166]

---

164. "Prescription for Trouble: Using Antibiotics to Fatten Livestock," Union of Concerned Scientists, 2013, http://www.ucsusa.org/food_and_agriculture/our-failing-food-system/industrial-agriculture/prescription-for-trouble.html.

165. "Beef Production," US EPA, 2015, https://www.epa.gov/sites/production/files/2015-07/documents/ag_101_agriculture_us_epa_0.pdf.

166. See "Chapter 6: Soy, Corn & Water" for a detailed description of no-till planting.

"Sure enough, year by year the steaks were getting better. Eventually the New York strip won best meat product in Georgia. We went from having to spit it out to winning an award."

I'm ready to congratulate Kristan on their top honor, but a sting in my sandal requires my attention. Without missing a beat, Kristan bends down and scoops fire ants off my toes. She is my cowbird. She yells over to Forrest, who busied himself removing fallen logs off the fence rails. It's time to get back in the Pioneer and introduce me to the pigs.

"How did you get in the business of raising pork?" I ask back inside the Pioneer. The engine growls.

"We started raising beef for our family alone, but people showed up at the farm wanting to buy. All of a sudden those people were telling other people, and we would have two to three families a week showing up. People would go in together and buy a whole cow. Then those same people asked if we could raise pastured pork. They wanted pigs that didn't grow up on concrete and didn't get their tails clipped."

A common pig "vice" among swine warehoused together in overcrowded pens is tail biting. This favored pastime for confined pigs causes infections and abscesses, putting the meat at risk for rejection for human consumption at the slaughter house, a costly designation for the pig owner.[167] Experts on pig behavior suggest the need for "enrichment"—in other words things like, hay bedding, mud, more room, possibly a peek at the great outdoors, but instead piglets' tails are clipped with scissors (without anesthesia), teeth are pulled, and a steady stream of antibiotics is fed to swine to keep them healthy enough to be edible.[168]

The Pioneer stops. Pigs are clustered in the shade of the woods. A few large ones stretch themselves lazily in the mud.

---

167. "Carcase condemnation terms," Queensland Government, Department of Agriculture and Fisheries, 2009, https://www.daf.qld.gov.au/animal-industries/pigs/pig-health-and-diseases/disease-prevention/carcase-condemnation-terms.

168. "Improving Pig Welfare: Addressing Tail Docking," The Pig Site, 2015, http://www.thepigsite.com/articles/5123/improving-pig-welfare-addressing-tail-docking.

"Eww-wee," Kristan yells. The pigs turn their heads in our direction. "It makes me sad to call them over without food." Her voice is full of emotion. She playfully scolds her son for not remembering the bread. "Forrest, call some more over here."

Forrest yells out and repeats, "Sue-wee," stretching the "e" long like taffy. Dozens of pigs run toward the fence.

"Pigs love being in the woods. With their snouts they dig, get grubs, and look for acorns. They eat persimmons that fall from the trees. It's all super good food for pigs. Our pigs are allowed to be pigs."

"Do you rotate the pigs onto a different pasture?"

"We have three permanent areas for pigs. They don't rotate because they are not herbivores. They're omnivores like chickens."

Only 3 percent of pigs raised in the US live on pasture. The other 97 percent live a very different existence. Unlike cattle, which spend part of their lives outdoors before intensive feeding, nearly all 100 million hogs raised in the US live their entire lives indoors in small pens.[169] The mama pigs live in gestation crates, similar in design to a shopping cart without the wheels. Slatted floors catch their abundant excrements. One building of 500 hogs expels 5,100 gallons of waste every seven days. In one year, all swine in confinement release enough manure and urine to fill 77,000 Olympic-size pools.[170]

The pigs oink, snort, and wait to be fed. "I'm sorry, guys, we don't have any bread," says Kristan. "I'm sorry," she says again. The pigs grunt in disappointment and walk back to the mud and the shade of the trees. The piglets trail behind their mamas.

"We started raising pigs around the same time we began selling beef to Whole Foods," she says. "The buyers from the Savannah Whole Foods

---

169. Barry Estabrook, *Pig tales: an omnivore's quest for sustainable meat* (New York: W.W. Norton & Company, 2015).

170. "Swine Manure Management Planning, ID-205," Purdue University Cooperative Extension Service *and Indiana Soil Conservation Service,* 1999, https://www.extension.purdue.edu/extmedia/id/ID-205.html. The total is based on fifty-one billion gallons of manure generated.

came to our farm and said they were tired of people coming to the store and asking why they didn't have Hunter Cattle meat products. When Whole Foods told us how much meat they need, we knew we alone couldn't provide those quantities. That's when we thought about partnering with other local farms. The meat scientist was our first partner. Our first pork partner was an old man who was selling off all his pigs and equipment. My dad called him to ask him why: 'We thought you loved farming.' The farmer told Dad at auction he was getting the same price for his pasture-raised pig as a pig coming off a feedlot. We told him if he continued farming, we'd buy all his animals at a higher price."

The cooperative model of partnering allows farms to remain small, yet access traditional distribution channels. This is in stark contrast to the vertical integration model dominating the meat industry.[171] In a vertical integration model, a corporation owns the entire supply chain. Contract farmers own the property and machinery, care for animals as instructed by the company, and are responsible for managing the waste. Contract farmers do not set prices for animals. Payment is rendered upon the delivery of edible animals. So while the farmer has no control over the method of animal husbandry, he/she assumes all the risk.[172]

"We sell only to smaller natural food stores because they understand they can't buy a whole bunch of tenderloins or rib eyes directly from small-scale farms. We have a whole cow you need to buy. We've turned away big-name grocery chains wanting to sell our meat. They want the meat for cheap, leaving us very little profit. They don't care if they put us out of business in two years because they worked us to death."

Forrest drives us to the MooMa's Farm Store, the family market. The store sells Hunter Cattle meat and local food products from neighboring farms.

---

171. See "Chapter 9: Dairy & Water" and "Chapter 11: Chocolate & Water" for further discussion of cooperatives.
172. Barry Estabrook, *Pig tales*.

"The farm store was my mom's idea," says Kristan. "Me, my dad, and my brothers told her no one is going to drive out here to the middle of the woods to buy food. She did it anyway. And sure enough, people come out. And as more people came they asked us if they could host birthday parties and weddings out here. But the best part is offering educational tours to our visitors."

Forrest returns from inside the store with carbonated juice drinks. He puts an icy-cold glass bottle against his flushed cheeks. I do the same.

~

"We bring the kids here to the hen house to collect eggs." I walk with Kristan and Forrest into the area designed for tours. "It's common for kids to ask why eggs are not with the rabbits. Adults also have surprisingly limited experience with farm life. I've explained to grown women that the boars do not have tumors, those are their balls, their testicles," she adds for emphasis. I nearly choke on my fizzy drink.

"Kids think eggs are made in factories," says Forrest, who walks with us unfazed by his mother's language.

"In many ways the kids are correct," I say.

"You are right. So much food is made in a factory."

Livestock in America is overwhelmingly raised in the factory setting of an AFO. Overall, 94 percent of poultry, pigs, and cattle spend all or part of their life on a feedlot or in a confined structure off pasture.[173]

"When people visit our farm," Kristan tells me, "we use the opportunity to talk about why it is important to know where your food comes from. Once people understand how we raise animals, they know why

173. Nil Zacharias, "It's Time to End Factory Farming," *Huffington Post*, 2011, http://www.huffingtonpost.com/nil-zacharias/its-time-to-end-factory-f_b_1018840.html. Ninety-four percent is the average for AFO/CAFO-raised chicken (broilers and egg-layers), turkey, pigs, and cattle. Seventy-eight percent of all cattle and 99.9 percent of chickens raised for meat raised and sold in the US are from an AFO/CAFO.

it costs more. Like, did you know it takes two years to raise a grass-fed cow?" She turns to look at me. "That's one year longer than a cow finished on grain in a feedlot."

"Why would a farmer finish the cow with grain and corn instead of keep them on the pasture?" I ask.

"Because it puts more weight on the animal faster, getting a higher price."

The water footprint of a 1,000-pound animal is 1.8 million gallons of virtual water. Ninety-eight percent of the water footprint of an animal is from what it eats. While animals finished on grain and corn are raised up to a year faster than the exclusively grass-fed livestock, the water footprint totals are five times larger for the confined or feedlot animals. The difference is water-intensive corn. Each year 6 trillion gallons of *blue* water from reservoirs, lakes, rivers, and aquifers is applied to American corn fields alone.[174]

"A guy called the MooMa Store and asked how much our rib eye costs. '$18.99 a pound,' I said. 'What in the world?' the man said. 'I can find rib eye for $9.99 a pound at the grocery store. You're probably not selling much,' he continued. I told him we're selling out every week. 'People must make way more money than me,' he said. I told him I don't think that's the case. People would rather eat meat once a week instead of twice a week. I spent ten minutes on the phone with him. I went on to tell him the difference in how the meat animal is raised and how it leads to better health for the animal, the land, and people who eat the meat."

"Did he end up coming into the store for the rib eye?" I ask.

"When our conversation was done he told me, 'I'll be seeing y'all tomorrow.'"

---

174. Mesfin M. Mekonnen and Arjen Y. Hoekstra, "A Global Assessment of the Water Footprint of Farm Animal Products," *Ecosystems* 15, no. 3 (April 2012), http://link.springer.com/article/10.1007/s10021-011-9517-8. Ninety-eight percent of the 1.8 million gallons of virtual water embedded in a 1,000-pound animal comes from what it eats. In the US, four out of every ten acres of corn is grown for livestock feed.

Americans eat ninety-eight pounds of red meat (beef, pork, lamb), and an additional seventy pounds of poultry (chicken and turkey) each year, more than any other country.[175] In the seven decades since 1950, the American diet has increased by thirty-four pounds of meat, largely due to a drop in meat prices from the proliferation of AFOs.[176] But we pay for the *external cost* of meat with diminished water quality and health, just not at the time of purchase.

Studies over the past three decades found grass-fed animals to have superior levels of Omega-3 fatty acids, vitamin E, beta-carotene, and conjugated linoleic acid (CLA).[177] The meat from grain-fed animals have higher levels of saturated, trans fat, and Omega-6 fatty acids.[178]

"People are willing to pay more when they understand how much more nutrition is in the food grown like we do. One little girl, after hearing me talk about the Omega-3s in our eggs, said, 'So I'd have to eat three store eggs to get as much nutrition as one of yours?' When you look at it from that stand point, you're getting better bang for your buck."

~

We move upstairs to the loft. Forrest leaves us to help his uncle with meat processing down below. The whirr of the floor fan on full blast is

175. "Agricultural Statistics 2015," USDA National Agricultural Statistics Service, 2015: XIII–5, https://www.nass.usda.gov/Publications/Ag_Statistics/2015/Ag_Stats_2015_complete%20publication.pdf. Totals are based on 2013 figures.

176. "Profiling Food Consumption in America," *Agricultural Fact Book*, USDA: 13–21, https://assets.documentcloud.org/documents/2461300/usda-chapter2.pdf. Our meat consumption increased from 159 pounds in 1950 to 1,93l pounds in 2013.

177. Cynthia A. Daley, et al., "A Review of Fatty Acid Profiles and Antioxidant Content in Grass-fed and Grain-fed Beef," *Nutrition Journal* (2010), https://nutritionj.biomedcentral.com/articles/10.1186/1475-2891-9-10.

178. An Australian study looked at three groups of meat: grass-fed, short-term rain-fed (80 days), and long-term grain-fed (150–200 days). The long-term grain-fed group was found to have higher levels of saturated, menstruate trans fat at Omega-6 fatty acids. The short-term grain-fed animals had similar levels of fat as the grass-fed meat but with significantly diminished levels of Omega-3s and CLA.

music to my ears. I make myself comfortable on the plaid couch draped with a crocheted afghan. A bible is placed on a wooden stand in the center of the coffee table.

"We started renting this space to overnight guests. Most people who rent up here just want to learn from us. And we are happy to teach them what we know," says Kristan.

"So this is like an incubator for organic livestock farmers," I say. I recall the organic vegetable incubator I visited near Seattle.

"I hadn't thought of it that way. But that is exactly what this has become," she smiles broadly. "Some people ask us, 'Why are you telling people how y'all do things? Aren't you increasing your competition?' What they don't understand is that all of us small family farms are on the same team up against the big dogs."

One million American farms have disappeared since 1950. As of 2010, four "big dogs," each with annual earnings in the billions, control 85 percent of the beef market, 65 percent of pork, and 51 percent of poultry.[179]

"If you feed an animal what they're supposed to eat, in an environment they're supposed to be in, it's better for the earth, for the animal, and for us who eat them. The more people spread the word, the more people like us can grow."

And grow they must.

---

179. "How Corporate Control Squeezes Out Small Farms," Pew Charitable Trusts, July 18, 2012, http://www.pewtrusts.org/en/research-and-analysis/fact-sheets/2012/07/18/how-corporate-control-squeezes-out-small-farms.

Managed Intensive Rotationally Grazed, Pasture-Raised Grilled Burgers with Homemade Organic Buns

Makes 4 servings

35 minutes to prepare

8 minutes to cook for medium burgers

I know the recipe name is a mouthful. But it is the only way I know how to differentiate the *best* beef from all the rest. The truth is, this is my second attempt at writing this chapter. My first attempt was called "Beef & Water" and based on a cattle ranch fifteen miles from my home. On that ranch, 150 cattle roamed freely on 3,500 acres of mountainous leased land. While there was much I loved about the ranch, including the father and son cowboys, there were things about it that just didn't seem right. It was an example of a farm that is *better* for water but not *best*.

In the first ranch, the cattle, unfettered by fencing, trampled all over the hillside of oak trees and native shrubs in search of food. The cow-to-acre ratio was 1:23 (one cow for every twenty-three acres). This ratio doesn't include another several hundred acres of pasture the cows are rotated through for half the year. Even with 200 miles of freeway separating both pastures, this farm is considered rotationally grazed. In fact, according to a USDA survey of grass-fed beef, the majority of pasture-based farms are rotationally grazed. But are they managed? Not in the way I saw at Hunter Cattle.

At this point you might be thinking, how in the world can I know all those things when I choose my meat? And my answer is, *How can we not?* On average, 27 percent of our total human water footprint results from our love of meat.[180] Too many ongoing environmental disasters of our time—water pollution, soil erosion, air pollution, deforestation, GHG emissions, dead zones, lowered ground tables—can be traced back to raising livestock.

At a restaurant I order like a vegetarian; on a good night I eat like a vegan, *unless* I trust the meat is coming from farms like Hunter Cattle. After I left Kristan and Forrest, I treated myself to a burger at Green Truck Pub in Savannah. The restaurant serves two types of burgers: vegan and burgers made from Hunter Cattle beef.

In my home kitchen, my meat is exclusively from small-scale pasture-based farms. The chickens and ruminant animals are rotated, and the pigs are allowed to be pigs in a paddock. I prefer to buy direct from ranchers at my local farmers' market so I can ask questions. Before I buy meat at a meat counter, I go home and study their website and call or email if I have more questions. Asking questions, lots of them, is the only way to know if a particular farm or label is the *best*. Each time we ask a question, we strengthen the movement for an overhaul of our current food systems. We let food producers know we are informed, and we care.

Managed, intensive, rotationally grazed, pasture-raised, and organic meat is more expensive per pound than the alternative because it reflects the actual cost. Our bodies don't need 270 pounds of meat a year. In fact, we don't need any at all.

Ingredients

1 pound beef for every four patties

Salt to taste

---

180. Arjen Y. Hoekstra, "The hidden water resource use behind meat and dairy," *Animal Frontiers* 2, no. 2 (April 2012): 3–8, http://waterfootprint.org/media/downloads/Hoekstra-2012-Water-Meat-Dairy.pdf.

Organic pepper to taste
Organic garlic powder to taste

Directions

1. Mix the ground beef with the spices to your taste. I mix with my hands. Let the meat sit for at least 20 minutes at room temperature to let the meat sit in the spices.
2. Hand-form the patties to ¾-inch thickness by rolling balls and slightly pressing them down in between your hands to make a disc shape. Place the patties on something flat like a baking sheet. Slightly indent the patties in the center with your thumb, top and bottom (this keeps them from rising into fat little patties on the grill).
3. I use the following guide for the grill time of patties:

   Medium-rare:

   Cook first side for 3 minutes, second side for 4 minutes.

   Medium:

   Cook first side for 3 minutes, second side for 5 minutes.

   Medium-well:

   Cook first side for 3 minutes, second side for 6 minutes.

   Well-done:

   Cook first side for 3 minutes, second side for 7 minutes.
4. Garnish the burger with organic cheese and local greens and vegetables. My favorite garnishes are grilled bell peppers and poblano chiles. My burger garnishes reflect the flavor of the season.

Homemade Organic Buns

Makes 8 large buns or 16 sliders

45 minutes to prepare

15 minutes to bake

Ingredients

2 cups warm organic milk*

¼ cup organic farm-fresh pastured butter, melted*

¼ cup warm water

¼ cup fair-trade sugar

2 (0.25 ounce) packages active dry yeast

2 teaspoons salt

6 cups unbleached organic dry-farmed or rain-fed white flour

**Purchase animal products from farms implementing a managed rotational pasture system (see "Chapter 9: Dairy & Water" for more information)*

Directions

1. Preheat oven to 375°F.
2. Stir together milk, butter, water, sugar, and yeast in a large bowl. Let it stand for 5 minutes.
3. Mix in the salt and flour gradually. Stir until the dough is supple.
4. Divide the dough in half, then quarters, then eighths (stop here if you want large buns). Separate one last time to sixteenths if you want smaller, slider buns. Form the dough into balls and

place on a baking sheet dusted with flour about 3 inches apart. Let the buns rise for 20 minutes away from drafts. I place the buns to rise in a cool oven.

5. Bake for 15 minutes. They should have a slight golden hue when done. Once cooled, slice the buns horizontally with a serrated knife. I freeze the extra buns (unsliced) for the next barbecue.

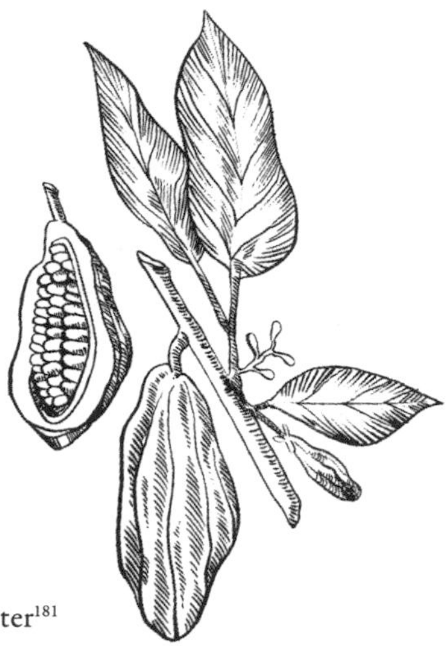

CHAPTER 11

Chocolate & Water

1 chocolate bar = 449 gallons of water

1 pound of chocolate = 7,727 gallons of water[181]

SWEET MEMORIES CLING to chocolate. As a child, I stood next to my mother as she grated the stone-ground Mexican chocolate into a pan. The chunky discs, individually wrapped, held the promise of cinnamon and sugar embedded in coarse dark cocoa. The gritty powder melted into the milk. The hot, fragrant *cho-co-la-te* served in *tazas*, clay mugs, and gulped down in a few swallows had close to 2,000 gallons of virtual water.

The water footprint of chocolate is four times larger than that of a pound of beef.[182] Cacao trees require between fifty to eighty inches of

181. Mesfin M. Mekonnen and Arjen Y. Hoekstra, "The Green, Blue and Grey Water Footprint of Crops," *Hydrology and Earth System Science* 15 (2011): 1577–1600, http://waterfootprint.org/media/downloads/Mekonnen-Hoekstra-2011-WaterFootprintCrops_1.pdf. Water footprint totals for a chocolate bar are based on 100 grams (3.5 ounces). The totals assume the chocolate to consist of 40 percent cocoa paste, 20 percent cocoa butter, and 40 percent cane sugar. Chocolate with a higher percentage of cocoa results in higher water footprint totals.

182. "Who Consumes the Most Chocolate," The CNN Freedom Project, January 17, 2012, http://thecnnfreedomproject.blogs.cnn.com/2012/01/17/who-consumes-the-most-chocolate. Americans eat eleven pounds of chocolate on average or 20.1 percent of the global consumption according to 2008/09 figures. Europeans eat the most, representing 49.3 percent of the global cocoa market. Based on these totals, the American chocolate water footprint equals 85,000 gallons of virtual, enough water to fill 1,000 bathtubs.

water annually to grow.[183] Cacao—chocolate in its raw form—is grown with 98 percent *green* water: rain.[184] But the water supply, both too much and too little from a shifting climate is growing too unpredictable for a growing number of the 5.5 million small farms growing 90 percent of world's cacao.[185] Drought and downpours stunt or spoil the harvest. Throughout the Cocoa Belt, trees are uprooted or burned to the ground and replanted with sturdier cash crops. On the Ivory Coast, the single largest cacao producer, rubber trees tapped for the latex oozing from the trunk like syrup are fast replacing cacao trees.[186] The current cacao shortage of one million tons is expected to worsen.[187]

I sit across from Alex Whitmore, co-founder of Taza, in the boardroom.[188] He sits upright, slender and tall. His formal manner contrasts with his work attire of shorts and a t-shirt. Alex was introduced to Meso-American stone-ground chocolate as an anthropology major. Years later he apprenticed with a *molinero*, a miller of cacao beans, in Oaxaca, Mexico.[189]

---

183. The "Cocoa Belt" is the tropical climate within twenty degrees of the equator in both directions.
184. Mekonnen and Hoekstra, "The Green, Blue and Grey Water Footprint of Crops." You can find this study as well as a short summary of chocolate water totals at the Water Footprint Network website found at http://www.waterfootprint.org.
185. "Fairtrade and Cocoa: Commodity Briefing," Fairtrade Foundation, August 2011, http://www.fairtrade.net/fileadmin/user_upload/content/2009/resources/2011_Fairtrade_and_cocoa_briefing.pdf.
186. "Ivory Coast reaps more rubber as farmers shift from cocoa," *Reuters*, February 13, 2013, http://www.reuters.com/article/rubber-ivorycoast-output-idUSL5N0BDB9S20130213. In 2012 the Ivory Coast exported 255 tons of rubber/latex. An output of 600,000 tons is targeted by 2020, a 40 percent growth rate.
187. Ganesh S. Vidhate and Rekha S. Singhal, "Extraction of cocoa butter alternative from kokum (Garcinia indica) kernel by three phase partitioning," *Journal of Food Engineering* 17, no. 4 (2013). You can find a comprehensive summary of this study at http://www.confectionerynews.com/Ingredients/Cocoa-butter-fat-replacers-are-progressing-but-more-work-needed-say-researchers.
188. Alex Whitmore in discussion with the author, June 2014.
189. "Cacao" is the bean from the cacao tree, scientific name *Theobroma cacao*. "Cocoa" is the bean after it has been processed.

Importing cacao beans from the Americas, he now brings the centuries-old tradition of Mexican chocolate making to his hometown of Boston.

Framed photographs of farmers posing next to cocoa trees hang from each of the boardroom's white walls. "How much lower are the yields of an organic compared to a conventional farm?" I ask while examining the photographs.

"Substantial. A farm using heavy chemical inputs can double its yield. That said, keeping the farm clean and the trees pruned and trimmed goes a long way in minimizing pests, fungus, and disease. So does the right balance of compost, sun, and shade."

The cacao tree naturally grows under the shade of the rainforest.[190] The heavy rainfall and humidity below the canopy of the forest sustained the trees for over 2,000 years.

In the twentieth century, the cacao tree was brought out of the shade and into the full sun. Farmers and scientists discovered cacao trees produce twice as many pods in full sunlight. This discovery came with a warning of "new dangers" resulting from lack of shade, such as invasion of weeds, degradation of soil, and new pests.[191] Seduced by the promise of higher yields, farmers cleared rainforests in the following decades.

Absent shade, yields increased.[192] So too has the use of agrochemicals to combat the new dangers. In regions of West Africa, the top grower of cacao, pesticide use doubled in the three years between 2007 and

---

190. "*Theobroma cacao* (cocoa tree)," Kew Royal Botanic Gardens, http://www.kew.org/science-conservation/plants-fungi/theobroma-cacao-cocoa-tree.
191. R. K. Cunningham, "What Shade and Fertilisers are needed for Good Cocoa Production?," *Cocoa Growers Bulletin*, no. 1 (1963): 11–16, http://orton.catie.ac.cr/repdoc/A7995i/A7995i.pdf.
192. K. Ofori-Frimpong et al., "Shaded versus unshaded cocoa: implications on litter fall, decomposition, soil fertility and cocoa pod development," Nature Conservation and Research Center, Ghana, http://www.academia.edu/6640169/Shaded_versus_unshaded_cocoa_implications_on_litter_fall_decomposition_soil_fertility_and_cocoa_pod_development.

2010 alone.[193] Worldwide, chemicals are relied upon to impede disease, fungus, and pests that can spoil 30–40 percent of annual harvests. New research finds the yields in medium-shaded trees to be almost twenty pods more per tree than unshaded trees.[194]

Latin America is the sweet spot for organic cacao production, representing 70 percent of the market share.[195] Acreage of organic cacao

---

193. George Afrane and Augustina Ntiamoah, "Of Pesticides in the Cocoa Industry and their Impact on the Environment and the Food Chain," in *Pesticides in the Modern World—Risks and Benefits*, ed. Margarita Stoytcheva (InTech, 2011), http://www.intechopen.com/books/pesticides-in-the-modern-world-risks-and-benefits/use-of-pesticides-in-the-cocoa-industry-and-their-impact-on-the-environment-and-the-food-chain. In Ghana, where agrochemicals are heavily subsidized, insecticide spraying alone more than doubled in the three-year period between 2007 and 2010. Mosudi B. Sosan et al., "Insecticide residues in the blood serum and domestic water source of cacao farmers in Southwestern Nigeria," *Chemosphere* 72, no. 5 (May 2008). In Nigeria, Diazon (a high toxicity pesticide) was found at "above acceptable levels" in the streams and wells (the primary source of drinking water) in villages where cacao is the primary industry. The same chemical coursed in the blood streams of 34 percent of farmers sampled. Residues were detected in all water tested from nine villages. Diazon was found in four out of the nine villages tested for this study.

194. Ofori-Frimpong et al., "Shaded versus unshaded cocoa." This study examines the gains reaped from the low-shade system. While unshaded cacao trees double yields in comparison to trees in heavy shade, 75 percent of the harvest was lost to disease, cherelle wilt (a plant affliction that causes young pods, cherelles, from ripening), and damage from rodents who nest in the cacao tree in the absence of other trees. The trees in medium shade, although they bloomed fewer cherelles, lost the least amount of harvest, with 35 percent. In the end, the trees in medium shade had twenty more healthy pods on average than the unshaded trees. The crop loss from the medium-shade was the least, at 35.4 percent, followed by the heavy-shaded trees at 57.2 percent. The unshaded trees had both the highest percentage of crop loss and the least amount of nutrients in the soil. When examining the mean number of total healthy pods, the medium-shaded tree had the highest with eighty healthy pods followed, by the unshaded with sixty-one, closely followed by the heavy-shaded cocoa at fifty-eight. This study was conducted on three farms in Ghana all within close proximity to each other to control for variance of temperature, rainfall and soil type. Three types of farms were studied: heavy shade, medium shade, and unshaded.

195. "A study on the market for organic cocoa," International Cocoa Organization, September 2006, http://www.icco.org/about-us/international-cocoa-agreements/cat_view/30-related-documents/37-fair-trade-organic-cocoa.html.

is growing worldwide, but the expansion is slow. As of 2012, only 0.5 percent of the world's harvest was certified organic.

"How many chocolate factories in the US are organic?"

"A small handful are 100 percent organic. The number grows if you include companies with organic capabilities, meaning one or more of their products are certified. Many more chocolate producers purchase rainforest-certified cacao, which is not organic, but is meaningful in protecting forests."

Rainforests are like mini-oceans. Moisture embedded in the leafy green canopy evaporates and forms clouds, impacting global rainfall.[196] The forests covered over 14 percent of the total land surface of the planet. Today, totals dropped to less than 7 percent.

In the forests of West Africa and the Congo, deforestation reduced rainfall by half. The Amazon alone, the largest rainforest in the world, is the source of one-fifth of the fresh water on the planet. Rainfall there is expected to diminish 21 percent by 2050 under current deforestation trends.[197]

Loss of rainfall extends beyond South America.[198] For example, the Sierra Nevada snowpack, the main irrigation source for the Central Valley of California and top producer of milk and produce in the nation, recedes with the Amazon rainforest.[199]

---

196. Plants release water into the atmosphere through a process called transpiration. In the tropics, each canopy tree can release about 200 gallons (760 liters) of water each year. The moisture helps create the thick cloud cover that hangs over most rainforests. Even when it's not raining, these clouds keep the rainforest humid and warm. This description and more information available at http://environment.nationalgeographic.com/environment/habitats/rainforest-profile.

197. D. V. Spracklen, S. R. Arnold, and C. M. Taylor, "Observations of increased tropical rainfall preceded by air passage over forests," *Nature* 489, no. 7415 (2012).

198. "Climate Change and the Amazon Rainforest," Amazon Watch, http://amazonwatch.org/work/climate-change-and-the-amazon-rainforest.

199. David Medvigy et al., "Simulated Changes in Northwest US Climate in Response to Amazon Deforestation," *Journal of Climate* 26, no. 22 (2013). Find an in-depth summary of this study online at http://www.princeton.edu/main/news/archive/S38/31/66M12/index.xml?section=topstories.

Cacao from certified agencies like Fair Trade and Rainforest Alliance comprised 6 percent of the total chocolate market share, but the demand is growing.[200] Three of the largest US-based chocolate manufacturers have committed to purchasing rainforest-certified cacao for all or part of their chocolate by 2020.[201] This, like similar certifications, provides technical support and training to farmers to improve yields while building the biodiversity of the tropical forests. Environmental sustainability certifications are positioned to be significant drivers of *re*forestation.[202]

Alex stands to lead me out into a spacious room divided by cubicle partitions. Many staff members opt to stand while they work in front of large Mac computer screens. They are young, spirited Bostonians, like Alex.

"How many people work for Taza?"

"We have fifty-four employees, most in our production team, the people who make our chocolate, where I'll be taking you next." I follow him down the steps. Alex sprints down with ease in his running shoes. I do my best to keep up with him in my heeled sandals.

---

200. "Study on the costs, advantages and disadvantages of cocoa certification," International Cocoa Organization, October 2012, http://www.icco.org/about-us/international-cocoa-agreements/cat_view/30-related-documents/37-fair-trade-organic-cocoa.html.

201. You can find articles about the partnerships with chocolate companies and Rainforest Alliance with the following links: http://www.hersheys.com/bliss/our-story/rainforest-alliance.aspx http://www.mondelezinternational.com/Newsroom/Multimedia-Releases/Kraft-Foods-Expands-Sustainability-Goals-to-Build-on-Success

202. Moshe Inbar and Carlos A. Llerena, "Erosion Processes in High Mountain Agricultural Terraces in Peru," *Mountain Research and Development* 20, no. 1 (2000). Cynthia Graber, "Farming Like the Incas," *Smithsonian Magazine*, September 2011, http://www.smithsonianmag.com/history/farming-like-the-incas-70263217. One encouraged technique is the ancient Inca practice of terraces, largely abandoned in conventional agriculture. The carved giant steps of terraced hillsides minimize soil erosion, flooding, and nutrient runoff. In Peru, the origin of the Inca civilization, researchers found no run-off from well-maintained, cultivated terraces during the rainy season. Terraces retain water during dry seasons or droughts—a common companion in the age of climate change.

Downstairs, we stop in front of a painting of a full-scale cacao tree on a brick wall. Pods grow directly from the trunk in colorful clusters.

Next to the tree is a drawing of a pod cut in half, exposing the milky contents.

"Ripe beans are white?"

"Yes. Most people don't realize chocolate is a fermented food, at least premium quality chocolate is. Fermentation and drying give the bean its familiar brown color."

The natural airborne yeast and bacteria eat away the sweet, sticky coating during the fermentation process. The alcohols, vinegar, and acids created during the fermentation seep into the bean and reduce its bitterness.

Alex hands me a hairnet to put on before we walk into the roasting area. He stretches the hairnet easily over his own short-cropped hair. I ungracefully shove my curls into mine. We slip into a room kept segregated from the rest of the facility. Inside, I understand why. The roar of machines and the strong roasting smell overpowers my senses.

We walk toward the roaster. It resembles an oversized pot-belly stove.

"The beans get roasted at 240 degrees for about forty-five minutes," Alex yells. The roasted beans are slightly larger than almonds. "Next, the winnow machine separates the shell from the cacao nib. Nibs are quite popular since they've been found to have even more health properties than dark chocolate." He reaches into a bucket and gestures for me to grab some nibs from his outstretched hand.

"Do people snack on these raw?" I ask before I place the kernel in my mouth.

"Nibs are eaten raw, sprinkled on ice cream and salads, baked in cookies . . . The ways to eat them are endless."

I'm relieved to exit the room back into the quiet hall. "Is it standard practice to start with raw beans?"

"Most chocolate factories purchase finished chocolate from large manufacturers. The manufacturers follow the chocolate makers' specific formulas and deliver the solution in a tanker. Bean-to-bar chocolate factories, like us, begin with the bean."

"About how many bean-to-bar chocolate factories operate in the US?"

"About seventeen, if you don't count the small craft guys who roast a ton or less a year."

Bean-to-bar chocolate makers circumvent the established supply chain and buy pods direct from farmers or cooperatives. The producer ensures a premium-quality bean to the maker's specifications, and farmers receive a premium price above the New York Board of Trade (NYBOT) price, in these direct relationships. Taza, in addition to premiums, guarantees a price floor.[203]

This security may hold the solution to keeping farmers from abandoning cacao even in the face of a growing demand for chocolate.[204]

We slip through another door. Inside, the air is dusted with cocoa powder.

"Do you ever tire of the chocolate fragrance?"

"I don't smell it anymore," Alex laughs. I take in a deep breath and taste the candied air.

The production team readies hundreds of glossy chocolate discs to be wrapped and packaged in boxes identical to those stacked on shelves

---

203. The volatility of the global cocoa markets serves financial insecurity to the farmer. In 2000, for example, the price of cocoa traded for $714 (US) a ton due to an oversupply of beans. In 2011, the market soared to $3,775, reacting to political instability in the Ivory Coast (the single largest producer), and a drop in supply caused by drought. Taza pays a minimum of $500 above the NYBOT price and has a price floor of $2,800.

204. Katy Barnato, "Future of the Chocolate Industry Looks Sticky." *CNBC*, March 24, 2016, http://www.cnbc.com/2016/03/24/future-of-the-chocolate-industry-looks-sticky.html. The expected shortage of cacao is one million tons. This is partially explained by an increased demand in China and India. It is also explained by the conversion of cacao farms into more lucrative cash crops or the abandonment of farming altogether.

around the room. Salsa music plays on a transistor radio. I fight the urge to dance while I follow Alex into the adjoining room.

"This is our grinding room." The frigid temperature eliminates any thoughts of dancing. "Cacao nibs are ground in the *Molinos*." The circular stones are hand-carved in the Taza factory, a skill Alex learned during his short apprenticeship with a *Molinero* in Oaxaca. "One stone rotates while the other remains static, and together they grind the nibs into a flowing paste. The *Molino* squeezes the paste, called cocoa liquor, from inside the nibs. The liquid paste is next mixed with raw cane sugar in the mixing tanks."

A tall stack of one hundred-pound bags of sugar is off to the side wall in the adjacent room. Each bag wears the Fair Trade label. "Are all your ingredients Fair Trade?"

"We purchase ingredients direct from the farmer whenever possible. Our cinnamon and vanilla come from Villa Vanilla, a sustainable organic spice farm in Costa Rica. Sugar, we purchase from a certified Fair Trade, organic company."

Cacao has a long history of child labor abuses including human trafficking of children to work on farms. Socially responsible trade programs prohibit child labor and require fair wages.[205] In exchange, the certified farms are awarded price premiums and price floors. While Fair Trade is not an organic certification, additional requirements include minimized pesticide use, reduction of green house gases, and a ban on

---

205. Human trafficking of children on cacao farms has been studied more extensively in Africa. In the Ivory Coast and Ghana for example, 50 percent of children living in agricultural households work. Find an in-depth discussion, statistics, gains, and challenges to combat child labor and slavery at "Oversight of Public and Private Initiatives to Eliminate the Worst Forms of Child Labor in the Cocoa Sector in Côte d'Ivoire and Ghana, " Payson Center for International Development and Technology Transfer Tulane University, September 30, 2010, https://www.dol.gov/ilab/projects/summaries/2010CocoaOversightReport.pdf.

untreated waste water disposal.[206] Some individual chocolate producers develop their own socially responsible trade programs. Taza's is called Direct Trade.[207]

A few steps away is my favorite machine thus far. Liquid chocolate flows from a steel spigot.

"This machine both tempers and deposits the chocolate into molds," Alex tells me. "Chocolate needs to be tempered because cacao is half cocoa butter which solidifies at room temperature."

Tempering gives chocolate its sheen, snap, and a higher melting point. But it's unnecessary when palm oil is substituted for cocoa butter.[208] Confectioners favor the versatility and low price of palm oil. The replacement of cocoa butter with palm oil is expected to continue as farmers leave cacao farming.[209]

To produce the world's most popular vegetable oil, orderly rows of palm trees engulf tropic landscapes.[210] The metamorphosis of terrain is the most drastic in Indonesia.

---

206. "Study on the costs, advantages and disadvantages of cocoa certification," International Cocoa Organization, October 2012, http://www.icco.org/about-us/international-cocoa-agreements/cat_view/30-related-documents/37-fair-trade-organic-cocoa.html. You can also visit the Fair Trade website for more information on requirements at http://www.fairtradeusa.org

207. Taza's Direct Trade is third-party certified by Quality Certification Services, a USDA-accredited organic certifier.

208. "Cocoa butter fat replacers are progressing, but more work needed, say researchers," *Confectionary News*, July 10, 2013.

209. Ganesh S. Vidhate and Rekha S. Singhal, "Extraction of cocoa butter alternative from kokum (Garcinia indica) kernel by three phase partitioning," *Journal of Food Engineering* 117, no. 4 (2013).

210. "Oilseeds World Markets and Trade," USDA Foreign Agricultural Service, January 2014, http://apps.fas.usda.gov/psdonline/circulars/oilseeds.pdf. Palm oil is the most consumed oil in the US. In 2013, 34 percent of oil consumed was palm oil, followed by soybean oil at 27 percent. Two hundred fifty-five million metric tons of palm oil were consumed during the five-year period between 2008 and 2013. Palm oil can be found in over half of all packaged foods. In addition, palm is a biofuel and is used in cosmetic and cleaning products. For statistics on domestic palm oil consumed in comparison to all other oils, see the USDA report.

Indonesia is a gathering of 18,000 islands on the Indian Ocean, lush in biodiversity and host to one of the most extensive peatlands. Peatland is layers of soggy plant debris that act as freshwater reservoirs. Formed over 10,000 years, the layers of plant material can reach depths of seventy feet. This saturated land filters the water for animals and humans living downstream.

Peatlands are critical in regulating global climate. They hold 30 percent of the world's carbon, more than all the forests combined. Over the ages, peatlands absorbed 1.2 trillion tons of carbon dioxide, an amount equivalent to the carbon emitted from 34,000 coal plants in a year.[211]

Two million palm plantations grow on former peatlands in Indonesia. Illegal fires down virgin forests, draining the peatlands of fresh water to make way for palm crops.[212 213] The damage to the peatlands to clear the terrain for palm is irreversible. When drained and burned, carbon—the leading contributor to climate change—is released into the

---

211. For an extensive study on peatlands around the world and in Indonesia I looked to the following scholarly book and study: F. Parish et al., eds., *Assessment on Peatlands, Biodiversity and Climate Change: Main Report* (Kuala Lumpur: Global Environment Centre, and Wageningen: Wetlands International, 2008). Krystof Obidzinski et al., "Environmental and Social Impacts of Oil Palm Plantations and their Implications for Biofuel Production in Indonesia," *Ecology and Society* 17, no. 1 (2012).

212. "Unspontaneous Combustion: Forest Fires Record Levels of Air Pollution; and the End Is Not in Sight," The Economist, June 2013, http://www.economist.com/news/asia/21580154-forest-fires-bring-record-levels-air-pollution-and-end-not-sight-unspontaneous.

213. Five percent of the world's palm oil production is Roundtable on Sustainable Palm Oil (RSPO) certified. About 48.2 percent of the world's current RSPO-certified sustainable palm oil production capacity comes from Indonesia, followed by 43.9 percent from Malaysia, and the remaining 7.9 percent from Papua New Guinea, Solomon Islands, Thailand, Cambodia, Brazil, Colombia, and Ivory Coast. While the RSPO has begun to tighten regulations of certified members on the issue of deforestation and peatland conversion, as of 2013 a ban of such practices had not been implemented. For more information about the current rules and vision of the RSPO visit www.RSPO.org. For a discussion of current weaknesses of the RSPO certification in its protection of forests and peatlands go to http://www.greenpeace.org/seasia/Global/international/publications/forests/2013/Indonesia/RSPO-Certifying-Destruction.pdf.

atmosphere. In Southeast Asia, the biggest producer of palm oil, annual carbon dioxide emissions from peatland drainage is 650 million metric tons with an additional 1.4 billion released from peatland fires.[214]

~

Papel picado, paper cut into elaborate designs, depict the chocolate-making process. The bright orange, red, and yellow of the delicate paper hanging from the ceiling of the retail shop matches the walls in the room. Track lights illuminate the chocolate.

Alex searches the shelves for his favorites. He hands me *mole.* "Organic is cleaner for the river," he says. "The communities where we purchase our cocoa use the river for everything, to swim and bathe in and drink." It is estimated, 70 percent of chemicals applied to cacao are retained in the soil and washed into streams and rivers.[215]

"When companies like us pay a premium for organic cacao, these farmers don't need to make a difficult decision between polluting their river and making a living."

---

214. F. Parish et al., eds., *Assessment on Peatlands, Biodiversity and Climate Change: Main Report* (Kuala Lumpur: Global Environment Centre, and Wageningen: Wetlands International, 2008).

215. Ayinde Idris et al., "Analysis of Pesticide Use in Cocoa Production in Obafemi Owode Local Government Area of Ogun State, Nigeria," *Journal of Biology, Agriculture nd Healthcare* 3, no. 6 (2013): 1–9, http://worldcocoafoundation.org/wp-content/files_mf/1383602173Idris2013DiseasesPestsPesticideUse.pdf.

Taza Hot Chocolate

Makes 2 Servings

The Mexican hot chocolate tradition continues with my children. When they were babies, I held their tiny hands within mine and rubbed them together like they held the wooden handle of a *molinillo*, a chocolate whisk. We sang a Spanish nursery rhyme about chocolate.[216] Now, we drink hot chocolate on rainy days. When the kids see the first raindrops, they squeal for hot chocolate. But unlike that of my youth, the chocolate served in my house is organic, Direct Trade, and without palm oil.

Ingredients

2 cups organic milk (you can swap out the milk with organic soy, almond milk, or water)
1 Taza Chocolate Mexicano 2.7 oz. package (any flavor)
Pinch of salt (optional)

Directions

1. Chop or grate the chocolate and set aside.
2. Heat milk or water in a small saucepan over medium heat to just below a simmer.

216. Here are the words to the Spanish nursery rhyme. Try this with a favorite child. It is guaranteed to fetch giggles. *Uno, dos, tres-cho. Uno, dos, tres-co. Uno, dos, tres-la. Uno, dos, tres-te. Cho-co-la-te, cho-co-la-te, ba-te, bate cho-co-la-te.*

3. Remove the milk from the heat and add a pinch of salt.
4. Mix in chocolate. Stir frequently with a wooden spoon until the chocolate melts.
5. Return the pan to the stove and re-warm over low heat.
6. Froth the chocolate with a whisk or *molinillo* while the chocolate warms.
7. Remove from heat when chocolate is hot and frothy. Serve in your favorite *taza*.

Taza Chocolate Mexicano Cookies

Makes 24 cookies

15 minutes to prepare, longer if you use a double broiler to melt the chocolate

10 minutes to bake

Ingredients

2 Taza Chocolate Mexicano 2.7 oz. package (any flavor)
¾ cup all-purpose organic flour (preferably dry farmed)[217]
½ tablespoon organic ground cinnamon
¼ tablespoon baking powder
1 cup fair-trade organic sugar
¼ cup organic butter*
1 large organic egg*
1 teaspoon organic vanilla extract

**Purchase animal products from farms implementing a managed rotational pasture-based system. (see "Chapter 10: Meat & Water," "Chapter 9: Dairy & Water," "Chapter 7: Eggs & Water" for more information)*

Directions

1. Preheat oven to 350°F.
2. Place chocolate in a small glass bowl and microwave on high for 1 minute until almost melted. Or melt in a double boiler and stir often until nearly melted.

217. See "Chapter 1: Wheat & Water" for more on dry-farmed flour.

3. Combine flour, cinnamon, and baking powder in a medium bowl.
4. Cream sugar and butter together in a separate bowl. Add egg and beat well. Next, add cooled chocolate and vanilla and beat until just blended.
5. Add flour mixture into wet ingredients and blend.
6. Drop spoonfuls of dough on a greased or lined cookie sheet.
7. Bake for 10 minutes or until cookies almost set.
8. Remove from oven and let cool on cookie sheet for an additional 2 minutes.
9. Transfer cookies to wire rack. I serve with a scoop of organic chocolate or vanilla ice cream.

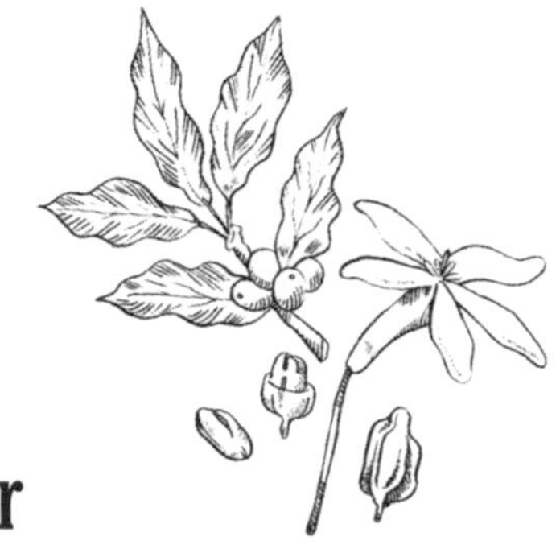

CHAPTER 12

Coffee & Water

1 cup of coffee (1½ tablespoons ground coffee) = 34 gallons of water[218]

1 pound roasted coffee beans = 2,270 gallons of water[219]

CAFE ARABICA GROWS beneath the regal Koa tree on the Hawaiian Cloud Forest Coffee farm on Mauna Kea, a dormant volcano on the Big Island. Moss and silver lichen enfold the trunk of the Koa in patches. The sinewy branches reach into a wide embrace constructing a canopy of leaves and sticks, capturing rain and moisture like a sticky spider web. Coffee needs high elevation, a temperate climate, and upwards of sixty inches of rain to flourish. The state of Hawaii is the only place in the United States that meets those requirements.

"Coffee is an understory tree," says Erik Gunther, co-owner of the coffee farm with his wife Hillery. "In the shade, the yield decreases but the fruit is bigger, lusher, and produces better quality." Like with the cacoa tree, the temptation of higher yields from *sun*-grown coffee is strong. The environment pays the price for higher yields with the clearing of forests, loss of biodiversity, and an increase of chemicals that make coffee the third most heavily sprayed crop in the world behind cotton and

218. M. M. Mekonnen and A. Y. Hoekstra, "The green, blue and grey water footprint of crops and derived crop products," *Hydrology and Earth System Sciences* 15 (2011): 1577–1600.
219. Ibid.

corn.[220] Organic coffee is *better* for water, but Eric and Hillery are my guides to understanding how organic shade-grown is *best*.

Lines of Koa trees follow the soft curve of gentle slopes on the Cloud Forest property. Erik and Hillery have planted 4,000 trees on their eighty acres thus far.

"The shade trees provide habitat for birds and insects," says Hillery.

Hawaii is habitat to 10,000 unique species of plants, insects, and fauna, but nearly 60 percent are in danger of extinction. "We know of four endangered species who visit us on this property. The Hawaiian hoary bat, Hawaiian duck, Pueo Hawaiian Owl and 'io hawk are frequent visitors to our property. But many species struggle on the islands. Trees are slowly dying, and no new trees are taking their place," says Hillery. "There are some state and federal lands replanting native trees, but their budget is too small to make much of an impact."

We stand near the coffee mill constructed of cedar and tin. Pieces of clouds remain low on the ground, a common feature at 2,500 feet above sea level. I ask about the extensive groves of eucalyptus trees lining the road up the mountain.

"The land planted with eucalyptus was once sugar cane land," Erik explains. "The trees are harvested and shipped to China. If you fo down to the harbor you'll see thousands of piled logs are ready to be loaded onto a ship."

"Were locals in favor of the conversion of sugar land to eucalyptus groves?"

"No, locals wanted the land planted with fruit or vegetables," says Hillery.

"Instead we grow wood for export," says Erik. "The wood eventually returns to the US as pallets and cardboard boxes packed with Chinese-made merchandise."

---

220. "Bitter Brew: The Stirring Reality of Coffee," Food Empowerment Project, http://www.foodispower.org/coffee.

"The state of Hawaii also grows seed for export. Genetically modified corn seed has surpassed all other crops," says Hillery.

The state of Hawaii imports 88 percent of its food, where it once was self-sufficient. Today 8,000 acres are planted with food crops on the islands, in comparison to 25,000 acres of corn and soy grown by five of the six largest agrochemical companies. Hawaii is the nation's largest testing ground for genetically modified (GE) crops, stressing waterways and diminishing the water-holding capacity of the land. Hawaiian grown GE corn was found to use seventeen times more "Restricted Use" insecticides than mainland field corn.[221] On the "Garden Isle" of Kauai, one agrochemical company applied ninety different chemicals to their test fields over a six-year period, spraying fields 243 days per year.[222]

"Eucalyptus trees are not part of the forest," says Erik. "When you take away native trees and plants, you take away the sponge that captures rain and moisture, keeping the rivers and gulches running year long."

Tropical forests act like above-ground lakes, critical to watersheds, pulling moisture from passing clouds. The multi-layered tropical forest of tall canopies, secondary trees, shrubs, fern layers, ground-hugging mosses, and leaf litter are responsible for capturing water by as much as 30 percent above the annual rainfall. Today, more than half of tropical forests have been destroyed worldwide.[223] Two-thirds of the original Hawaiian forest have vanished.[224]

The late nineteenth century marked the height of forest destruction on the Hawaiian archipelago. Hundreds of thousands of acres of

---

221. The five agrochemical companies testing in Hawaii are Monsanto, DuPont-Pioneer, Syngenta, Dow Chemical, and BASF. "Restriced Use" chemicals are not available to the general public due to their "potential to cause unreasonable adverse effects to the environment and injury to applicators or bystanders without added restrictions."
222. Bill Freese and Alexis Anjomshoaa, "Pesticides in Paradise Hawai'i's Health & Environment at Risk," Hawai'i Center for Food Safety, May 2015, http://www.centerforfoodsafety.org/files/pesticidereportexecsum_final-july-14-2015_21537.pdf.
223. "Bitter Brew: The Stirring Reality of Coffee," Food Empowerment Project, http://www.foodispower.org/coffee.
224. "Hawaii tropical moist forests," World Wildlife Fund, http://www.worldwildlife.org/ecoregions/oc0106.

native forest were cleared for agriculture and pasture. The destruction was halted only with the establishment of the forest reserve at the urging of sugar barons who understood that without forests there would be no water for growing sugar.[225] Hawaii's native forests are again under attack. The need for protection of forested watersheds intensifies, but a meager 1 percent of Hawaii's general fund is allocated to manage marine resources *and* 1 trillion acres of land.[226]

"We have plenty of big gulches, rivers, and waterfalls. The old timers said the big gulches and waterfalls along the Hamakua Coast were always running. Now they only run when it rains hard," says Hillery.

We walk the short distance from the entrance of the mill to a grove of coffee trees dwarfed by the mature Koas. I'm easily taller than the Cafe Arabica trees that were recently cut back.

"Every fifth year we cut back the coffee trees. It's a standard practice to maintain healthy yields. At this elevation it takes longer for the trees to regrow," says Erik.

"Does the slow growth affect the quality of the beans?" I ask.

"You've heard of mountain-grown coffee in Columbia?" Erik asks.

I nod my head. "The night temperature drops like here, to the low-fifties and sometimes high-forties. The cooler temperature slows down the time between flowering and harvest by two to three months."

"The bean has more time to develop its flavor. We think it's why customers who normally get upset stomachs from drinking coffee don't experience it with ours, because it doesn't have an acidic bite," says Hillery.

"The flavor is softer, smoother, more chocolaty than other varieties," says Erik. Hillery smiles at her husband's description, while my interest in taking a sip intensifies.

"When do you harvest?"

---

225. "Last Stand: The Vanishing Hawaiian Forest," The Nature Conservancy, 1989. http://www.nature.org/media/hawaii/the-last-stand-hawaiian-forest.pdf.
226. Ibid.

"We harvest daily," answers Erik. "Larger farms harvest by machine; our beans are hand-picked. It takes two to three weeks to harvest all the ripe coffee cherries. And then the process begins again." Mechanical harvesters, introduced onto coffee farms in the 1970s, harvest quickly and require far less labor, but it is not selective between the ripe and unripe beans. Instead, the mechanical harvester strips the tree clean, lowering the price and quality of the coffee.

We approach a tree. Hillery plucks a cherry to show me up close. The color of skin, dark red. I examine the cherry and wonder aloud how they remove the skin to expose the two beans inside. For an answer, they guide me away from the trees and toward the wet room adjacent to the mill. The lofty building houses a patchwork of tanks, machines, pipes, and ladders leading to narrow metal platforms.

"We fill this tank with water and place the cherries in here, up to 2,000 pounds." He points to somewhere among the metal and plastic.

"What is your water source?" I ask.

"We have access to county water, but we haven't used a drop in the last two years. County water is runoff from the forests. Wild pigs and mongoose are in that area. We rather not drink or use that water for our beans. We catch water from all our rooftops into a 60,000 gallon tank that we use for everything on this farm. Ultraviolet light kills any bacteria."

I contemplate the simple beauty of eating and drinking foods made with water harvested from the rain that falls on your own land.

Erik continues, "The pump sucks the cherries and water from the tank and takes it up to that rectangular box." He directs my attention overhead. "The water comes back down and continues in a loop." My head follows his finger like a cat across the room. "Last the cherries are carried to the pulper, separating the green bean from the skin. The skin pulp becomes mulch."

Nothing wasted.

"After the wet room, the beans are next taken to the drying shed." Our next stop.

Inside the drying shed, a former orchid greenhouse, there are wide-screened tables three across, ten deep. Erik rakes the layer of beans in one long line to turn them. Finished, he repeats in the other direction. The metal teeth glide across the screen, the sound interrupted only by dove calls. "I do this every morning. It's become my daily meditation."

We hike up the short path that separates the drying shed from the mill. In the distance the top of Mauna Kea is shrouded with clouds. "I learned to ski on Mauna Kea when I moved here in the '70s." Hillery looks up toward the direction of the cloaked mountain top.

"There used to be snow on Mauna Kea year-round. They held ski races on the Fourth of July," Erik adds. "Those days are gone. We have no snow pack on Mauna Kea anymore."

"It's in the middle of winter, and we've only had a few sprinklings of snow," says Hillery.

"We keep close tabs on the weather. We measure the rainfall and record the high and low temperature each day," says Erik.

"Any trends?" I ask.

"It was much wetter in the '70s. From 1984 to around 2005 the average rainfall was about 115 inches. We had a ten-year stretch where the average dropped down to 60–70 inches. In the last two years rainfall increased to 134 inches, but the high rainfall is attributed to El Niño effects. We will wait and see if it continues."

"What do you think caused the decrease in rain and snow?

"We think it's climate change," says Erik. He looks over to Hillery. She nods in agreement.

Inside the mill our voices echo off the metal machines. "All these devices run off sunshine." He makes a sweeping gesture to the line of machines. "Sixty-three solar panels are on the roof of the mill."

"The dryers run off a generator, but it's rare we use them. Most of our drying is accomplished in the drying shed," says Hillery. We walk deeper into the mill.

Seven screens shake vigorously to separate the coffee beans. "This here is a huller," says Hillery, standing next to another machine. "It removes the parchment off the bean." The papery film becomes compost.

"After the huller, the beans are sorted." Erik reaches into a bag and pulls out a handful of green beans. He points to a large bean in the center of his palm. "The highest grade is the pea berries." He nudges the oblong-shaped bean that looks like two fused together. He moves to a different bean in his hand. "The second highest grade is the extra fancy. They're the biggest and have the fewest amount of defects. If the bean has too many defects, it's classified fancy." The difference is slight between the extra fancies and fancies for the untrained eye. "Prime is the lowest grade. They're smaller or broken bits and pieces. They fall through the seven screens."

"What do you do with the prime beans?"

"Have you heard of Kona blend?" Erik asks. "The rule is only 10 percent of the beans have to be Kona in a Kona blend; 90 percent can be from anywhere else in the world. Prime ends up in Kona blend. Ground, you can't see the difference. The difference is in the flavor."

"And in the price," adds Hillery. "A pound of Kona blend is one-third of the cost of pure Kona."

The roasting room is last to be explored. As soon as I enter, it becomes my favorite. The ethereal smell of freshly roasted coffee clings to the cedar walls. A long, rustic wood table occupies the center of the room, perfect for tastings.

In the corner of the room is a twenty-four-kilo roaster, gleaming silver and gold. "A roasting profile has been programmed into the computer to manipulate the temperature and air flows in the roaster," Erik says, moving near the computer panel.

"What is your favorite roast?"

"We prefer the medium roast with no cream or sugar," answers Hillery. "You can discern the subtle flavoring in the lighter roasts."

"How often do you roast?"

"About two or three times a month," says Hillery. "We want our monthly coffee subscribers to receive their coffee a week after roasting when it's fresh yet it's had enough time to de-gas."

"De-gas?"

"You shouldn't brew your coffee the same day you roast it, because of degassing of carbon dioxide." Hillery hands me a glossy bag of medium roast. "Roasted coffee beans release gases for a week or two after roasting. The holes in a coffee bag allow the gases to escape without letting any air in. Air causes coffee beans to go stale like bread left out on the counter."

"What do you think of K-Cups?" I wonder as I examine the holes on the top of the coffee bag.

"Coffee is more flavorful when freshly ground. But beyond our preference of coffee flavor, there's the issue of added waste," says Hillery. "There's a whole lot of garbage generated by those pods." The number of mostly non-recyclable single K-Cups sold in one year can wrap around the Earth's equator more than twelve times.[227]

"We think we're spending more for organic coffee, but in fact you pay more per cup with a K-Cup than when you buy a pound of our coffee. Depending on how you brew it, you can get anywhere between fifty to one hundred cups per pound of coffee. If you spend thirty dollars a pound on coffee plus the flat-rate shipping, you're brewing sixty cups at about sixty cents a cup. The average K-Cup is seventy-five cents a cup."

Next to the mill is the tree nursery with seedlings sprouted from fallen coffee cherries. Chickens underfoot ceaselessly search for bugs

---

227. James Hamblin, "A Brewing Problem: What's the Healthiest Way to Keep Everyone Caffeinated?," *The Atlantic*, March 2015.

nearby. These natural pest controllers remind me to ask about the pest management on this farm.

"Insects overall don't like coffee," answers Hillery. "Unlike humans, insects don't like caffeine. The exceptions are the coffee borer beetle and coffee leaf miner."

"For the USDA organic seal you must only use approved inputs," says Erik. "If we have any issues, we work from the list. Maybe it's the shade, the clouds, or the soil, but we typically have no pest issues."

Coffee is among the most chemically treated crops worldwide and spraying is expected to intensify with warmer global temperatures. Researchers of the borer beetle in Colombian coffee fields, the third largest producer behind Brazil, found for every 1.8°F increase in temperature, the coffee berry borer became 8.5 percent more infectious on average.[228] Additionally, researchers found warmer temperatures caused females to lay more eggs and burrow deeper into the cherry. Chlorpyrifos, diazinon, and cypermethrin are used against the beetle on conventional coffee lands. These agrochemicals are toxic to birds and fish when leached into waterways, and Chlorpyrifos (Dursban) has been linked to birth defects.[229]

Organophosphate insecticide, disulfoton, and methyl parathion are applied on conventional grown coffee to minimize damage from coffee leaf miner. Methyl parathion is categorized in the Dirty Dozen, a list compiled by scientists and researchers at Pesticide Action Network, as the most toxic pesticide to humans, wildlife, and fish. While these organophosphate insecticides are highly restricted in the United States

---

228. Erika Westley, "Spurred by Warming Climate, Beetles Threaten Coffee Crops," *Yale Environment 360*, August 2010, http://e360.yale.edu/feature/spurred_by_warming_climate_beetles_threaten_coffee_crops/2312.

229. J.D. Sherman, "Chlorpyrifos (Dursban)-associated Birth Defects: Report of Four Cases," *Archives of Environmental Health* 51, no. 1 (1996): 5–8, http://www.ncbi.nlm.nih.gov/pubmed/8629864.

and other industrialized nations, their use remains widespread in developing nations, where nearly all coffee is cultivated.[230]

"Why organic?" It is the same question I ask every farmer.

"We made the decision to eat organic in our late teens," answers Hillery. "Nearly everything we eat is grown without chemicals. So we wouldn't do this any other way."

"We firmly believe that one hundred years ago everything any human ate was organic. Conventional *was* organic. In the last century we've had this grand experiment where most of the food has been sprayed with glyphosate, the key ingredient of Roundup, which the WHO recently categorized as a carcinogen and is liberally applied to GM seed crops in the state of Hawaii," says Erik. "I have this fantasy that eventually there will be more people who demand organic than the other way. Farmers, if they want to stay in business, will have to be organic."

"Maybe it will happen in our lifetimes," says Hillery.

"Maybe," I say. We all look out to the Mauna Kea Mountain wrapped in clouds.

---

230. "Biomonitoring Summary: Methyl Parathion, Ethyl Parathion," Center for Disease Control and Prevention, https://www.cdc.gov/biomonitoring/Methyl_Eethyl_Parathion_BiomonitoringSummary.html.

How to Brew the Best Cup of Coffee

A great cup of coffee begins with the beans. Look for organic, hand-picked, shade-grown coffee. Research the farm practices to be sure farmers didn't replace original forest with non-native shade-grown trees, a practice that occurs in coffee-growing countries around the world. Seek growers who keep the original forests intact or are working to replant forests on previously deforested land.

Buy whole beans and grind your own. Coffee loses its quality immediately after grinding. It is best to grind as you go for every cup of joe.

Don't freeze your coffee, instead store beans in an airtight container. Glass canning jars or a jar with a seal work fine.

Use filtered water but skip the bottled water, (we've got enough plastic floating around the planet). Consider attaching a filtration system to your tap.

Ditch paper filters and opt for a reusable filter. Not only does this reduce waste, but the reusable filter doesn't alter or absorb the flavor, unlike paper.

Measure 1½ tablespoons ground coffee for every 6-ounce cup (2 tablespoons for 8-ounce mug). Adjust up or down according to your taste.

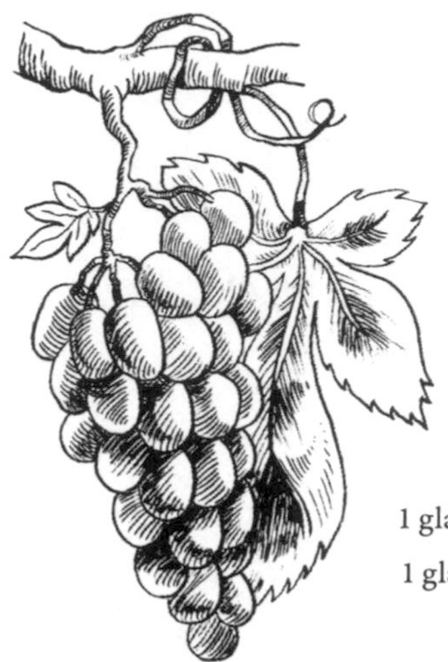

CHAPTER 13

Wine & Water

1 glass of white wine = 29 gallons of water

1 glass of red wine = 32 gallons of water[231]

WINE GRAPES PREFER to sip water. Plastic drip hoses snake between the lines of grapevines in warm wine regions of the US. In California, the fourth largest producer of wine in the world behind Italy, France, and Spain, 250 million cases sipped 1 trillion gallons of water from wells and rivers across the state in one year alone.[232]

Benziger Family Winery lured me to the small town of Glen Ellen in Sonoma Valley, California, a town with more grapevines than people. The vineyard is biodynamic. I meet with Mike Benziger, the visionary of the wine label and my tour guide into the complicated process of turning water into wine.[233]

We sit together on the brick patio between the wood Craftsman-style tasting room and a modern concrete production facility.

Overhead a crow and squirrel squabble in an oak tree.

---

231. Thomas Kostigen, *The Green Blue Book: The Simple Water-Savings Guide to Everything in Your Life (Emmaus, PA: Rodale, 2010).* Water footprint total is for a four-ounce glass of wine.

232. David Pierson, "Going Dry in a Sea of Wine: A Shrinking Water Table Pits Residents against Grape Growers," *Los Angeles Times*, September 2, 2013.

233. Mike Benziger in discussion with the author, May 2013.

"They're fighting over water," says Mike. We watch. The crow wins this time as the squirrel jumps away to a neighboring tree.

"Water is our biggest challenge. On this property, water is scarce and getting scarcer. It's April, and we've only had two and a half inches of rainfall. It could be the worst since 1850 when California began keeping weather records." Sonoma Valley is gripped by a drought that blankets 87 percent of the Western United States.[234]

"How many inches of rain do you receive on average?" I ask.

"Twenty-three, twenty-four inches."

"We knew this drought was coming, because we work with a long-term weather program. In anticipation, we began developing practices to drive our roots deeper. We apply less water and water later in the year. We adopted an innovative tool called 'electro conductivity mapping.'"

He takes out his smart phone from his back pocket to show me. A map of the farm appears on the screen. It's like a child's finger painting with blotches of different colors, but their map arrangement is far from the spontaneity of a preschool painting.

He points to different colors on the photo. "Each color signifies a soil geology. The red color code is a soil type that can hold more water. This blue region is drier and needs more water, and green represents soil with every quality."

"Do you irrigate less using these maps?"

"We can tailor our watering to the particular needs of each block. It also means we have better grape quality, because we pick the fruit at the height of perfection in each block; that of course leads to good wine." He tucks his phone into his pocket and leans back into the chair. The winery mirrors his relaxed style of understated elegance, like his combination of ironed khakis and sporty hiking boots.

---

234. Thirteen states are defined as the "West" according to the US Census. They are Alaska, Arizona, California, Colorado, Hawaii, Idaho, Montana, Nevada, New Mexico, Oregon, Utah, Washington, and Wyoming.

The sun burns away the early morning fog. The fresh scent of water lingers. Bees hover over lavender and roses in the garden near us.

"This farm teems with life," I speak louder to be heard above the chorus of bird calls in the trees shading the patio.

"It wasn't always the case. We hired the best consultant from Napa and the University of California to help begin our vineyard. Their technique was to control nature by eliminating it. The thought was grapes should have no competition, not from birds, insects, grass, weeds—zero. We eliminated everything with their recommended chemical dosages," says Mike.

Mike's first wine label was established in partnership with his wife and parents. In less than a decade, they built a winery label with a distribution of 2.6 million cases a year.[235] They were among the thirty largest wine producers in the United States. Today, the top thirty companies account for 90 percent of all wine sold, with the top three alone accounting for more than half.[236]

"We farmed for several years that way. You didn't see an insect or hear a bird. It was dead silent. We'd killed the property."

"What changed?"

"One day, my wife and I noticed the silence," he says. "It was our epiphany. Soon after we began the transition into biodynamics. It healed our farm. We doubled down when we discovered it improved the quality of wine."

Along with organic standards, biodynamics encompasses a framework designed to build biological diversity. When executed, the system

---

235. Lewis Perdue, "Requiem For a Legendary Brand: RIP Glen Ellen," Wine Industry Insight, http://wineindustryinsight.com/?p=46102. Glen Ellen Winery was founded in 1980 by Mike Benziger and his father Bruno. In 1982 the winery produced 7,000 cases and in 1988 sold 2.6 million cases. The label was sold in 2002 to The Wine Group (TWG) listed as the second largest wine producer in the US in 2012. TWG has since sold this label.

236. "Review of the Industry: The 10th Annual Ranking of the Largest Wine Producers in the United States," *Wine Business Monthly*, February 2013: 42.

is self-sufficient, requiring little to no external farm *inputs* such as fertilizers, seeds, and water.

We leave the patio and walk to the waiting tram parked on a dirt road. The electric vehicle transports guests on tours of the biodynamic vineyard. I'm the only guest, so I occupy the passenger seat next to Mike, the driver.

He drives the long, empty tram up to the ridge. From this vantage point, the property unfurls itself slowly like a good glass of wine. It is a collage of greens. Dark green spreads among the trees rooted in the soft slopes of hills. Light green of grape leaves shiver with the breeze. Mossy green crop cover sprouts between lanky vines tangled around strands of wire.

"We're inside a volcanic caldera sinkhole from an eruption thousands of years ago. For a winemaker, this is a candy store because of the diversity of soil types." He stops the tram and we slide out.

"Every plant, every grass planted here is by deliberate choice. Everything has a job. We are keen on biodiversity, but every plant also needs to make a contribution. A biodynamic farmer visualizes the property as a living organism. If you understand your property is alive, you have a powerful feeling of responsibility to care for it." His tone is infused with seriousness when he speaks about biodynamics.

Behind us is a soil probe. The slender pole stands quiet, sending wireless data about the soil moisture to a computer somewhere on this property.

"Computerized moisture probes are another technology we use to save water. The probes tell us where the moisture is and we can see where the roots are working. Every fifteen minutes the probes send data."

"How much water do you save using the soil probes?"

"They saved us 20 percent right off the bat. This is the third year using them. Once we delve in further with this technology we will save even more water."

Soil probes saves water yet the simple technology remains uncommon. This technology is found on only three out of every ten irrigated farms.[237]

"The probes help us know if the plant is in the right place."

"How does planting in the 'right place' save water?"

"When the rootstocks of the plant are adjusted to the soil, they make the least demand on the environment. For example, when you see one hundred acres of vineyards, only eighty acres should be farmed. It's the farmer's greediness to farm those twenty acres that takes 50 percent of the inputs like chemicals and water. Conventional agriculture gets impatient and borrows from the future to increase production today."

"Like borrowing water from the future?"

"Our farming methods regenerate the land. Instead of borrowing, we build biological capital like a bank account. We work off the interest. The funny thing is, when we place the least demand on the environment we grow the highest quality grapes."

"How many acres are planted with grapes?"

"Before we started biodynamics we farmed fifty-five acres of grapes on this property; now we farm thirty-five. We farm 245 acres biodynamically on five other locations. To produce 12,000 cases of wine a year, we buy additional grapes from forty growers."[238]

"Are the grapes you source from biodynamic farms?"

"Some of the farms transitioned from organic to biodynamic," Mike tells me. "We purchase from farms certified under the *Farming for Flavor* program we began in 2003. The 1,200 acres of grapes covered under this certification are organic," says Mike.

---

237. Chris Bertelsen (Agriculture Specialist, Spectrum Technologies, Inc.) in discussion with the author, September 2013. Spectrum Technologies is a company specializing in agriculture measurement information technology.

238. Benziger employs eighty full-time employees and seventy part-time employees, including family members. According to the Wine Institute, an industry advocacy group, Benziger is categorized as a small winery. The categories are determined by cases of wine produced.

Farming for Flavor regulates water usage. This is unlike the USDA Organic, the largest organic certification agency in the country.[239] No rules for water reduction are enacted in the USDA Organic guidelines. The certified farms near my home in Oxnard, California spray long, wide arches of water from sprinklers during the hottest time of the day when evaporation is at its peak. These same farms often irrigate during the rain.

Other third-party certifications suggest measures to reduce overall water usage on the vineyard and winery yet offer little to no protection of water quality. A third-party sustainability certification popular among many of the largest wine labels allows the use of chemical pesticides, herbicides, and synthetic fertilizers, universally recognized as water pollutants. A representative for this certification agency explained, pesticides and synthetic fertilizers are allowed as long as they stay out of waterways. Certain farming strategies can slow the movement of these pollutants, but chemical runoff will find waterways.

Mike leads me toward a deep ditch carved in the hillside. The earth is held in place with a rectangle of plexiglass. Printed on the plastic are the names of the soil types.

"These are the four layers of soil: topsoil, subsoil, regolith, and bedrock." The top two layers are thin, like dark chocolate cake that failed to rise.

"The green growth pretty much comes from the topsoil and subsoil. Roots grow in balls and stay in these top two layers." I see the tangled clumps of roots in the topsoil through the transparent Plexiglas. More prominent are the lanky roots' thickness of licorice winding deeper into the carved hillside.

"What we are trying to do is to get the bulk of our root systems that grow horizontal in the topsoil and subsoil to instead grow vertical into the bedrock and regolith layers."

---

239. Farming for Flavor is third-party certified by Stellar and is the organic farm of Demeter, the leading biodynamic certifier in the world.

"Why?"

"From a wine maker's perspective, the regolith and bedrock are the holy grail. Minerals are in those layers. If we can get our root systems to reach them, we can get flavors that shallow vines can't get."

"Do you water less with deeper root systems?"

"Much less—the plant draws moisture from the bottom two layers. We don't water during the hottest time of the year, from summer solstice to harvest time, when the grape ripens."

"On conventionally grown vineyards, do the root systems grow this deep?"

"No. Ninety-nine percent of the root is in the topsoil."

"Shallow roots lead to more water use," I say, making the connection between deep root systems and water conservation.

"Exactly right."

We walk along the rows of grape vines gripping the soft hills. The slight breeze carries perfume from the bloom.

"In December we had two big rain events," Mike says. "One rainfall in particular was so devastating it washed away every inch of road on this property. In the vineyards not a single speck of dirt moved."

"How is that possible?"

"The soil porosity, perfect. The soil tilt, perfect. The enzymes of the soil glue it together. The road, with no living activity to hold the soil together, washed away."

"What happened to your neighbors during the same storm?"

"They had erosion problems. It's what happened here before we became a biodynamic farm." He points to the steepest hillside. "After any good rain, the soil from the hillside covered the parking lot."

"And now?"

"Not a single soil particle moves. It's one of the real payoffs of green farming. It helps us get through extreme weather conditions."

Soil active with organic matter (SOM)[240] can better protect plants from drought conditions, pests, and disease. SOM builds and stores nutrients released into the plant, reducing or eliminating the need for commercial fertilizers. The soil becomes a sponge; minimizing runoff and flooding. If every acre of cropland was active with organic matter, soil erosion would drop by 72 percent.[241] It would save thirty-five billion dollars in soil every year and even more water.

"Are any of your grapes dry farmed?" I ask.

"Thirty percent."

Early California vineyards were commonly dry farmed. Plants grew exclusively with natural rain and moisture. While dry-farmed grapes are recognized as superior in flavor, they produce lower yields.[242] Modern grape growers favor irrigation for increased yields.

Dry-farmed grapes had been a longstanding tradition in Europe, thought to protect the "terroir" in each vintage, but the practice has become less common in Europe, too. France, the second largest wine producer in the world, was the last to lift the centuries-old ban on irrigation in 2006 in response to warmer global temperatures.[243]

Changes in climate will continue to increase the use of irrigation. A study published in the Proceedings of the National Academy of Sciences of the United States of America (PNAS) finds one quarter of current

---

240. "Soil Health Nuggets," USDA, National Resources Conservation Service, https://www.nrcs.usda.gov/Internet/FSE_DOCUMENTS/stelprdb1101660.pdf. Soil active with organic matter is simply soil alive with microbes and bacteria. One handful of soil contains more living organisms than there are people on the planet. These living organisms lie dormant unless fed carbon from plant and animal material and energy. When soil is healthy it is moist, dark—almost black in color with the scent of wet bark. It is the soil that thrives on Mike's small vineyard.

241. "Soil Organic Matter," USDA National Resources Conservation Service, October 2013, https://www.nrcs.usda.gov/wps/portal/nrcs/detailfull/soils/health/mgnt/?cid=nrcs142p2_053859.

242. See "Chapter 1: Wheat & Water" for an in-depth description of dry farming.

243. Jancis Robinson, "Irrigation Now Official in France," 2007, http://www.jancisrobinson.com/articles/irrigation-now-official-in-france. The four largest wine producers in the world in ranking order: Italy, France, Spain, US.

worldwide viticulture acreage will be characterized as "not suitable" for wine production by 2050. In California alone, the suitability of climate for viticulture is predicted to decrease between 50–63 percent by 2050. Present day wine grape growing regions will need more water to continue production, requiring misting to cool crops in the warmer summer temperatures and more water to control for frost damage in colder winters. Drills will continue to dig deeper for water, and rivers already suffering from lower flows will be tapped for more.[244]

We get back in the tram and descend the dirt road toward the ponds. On both sides of the tram, slow swaying grapes reach for the sky. Mike stops the tram.

"These are our recycling ponds," says Mike, pointing toward two ponds nested in the floor of a small valley. "All the industrial waste water from cleaning of the barrels, floors, and tanks comes down to this upper pond." We stand near the basin. "Gravity carries the water into this constructed wetland, what we call the living kidney because it removes the impurities of the water." Tall, thick papyrus and graceful calla lilies grow from the shallow water between the upper and lower ponds. "By the time the water moves from the upper pond to the lower pond, it's almost drinking-water quality."

"How is it possible?"

Mike reads my astonished expression. He is pleased, like a magician who produced a rabbit out of his hat to the amazement of the audience.

---

244. Lee Hannah et al., "Climate Change, Wine, and Conservation," Proceedings of the National Academy of Sciences of the United States of America, February 2013. Nine academics from universities around the world studied the impact of climate change on wine growing regions and the impact on water use and habitat loss resulting from the shifting of wine growing into new regions. Based on their models, a 25–73 percent in suitability is predicted for viticulture acreage around the world by 2050. In the US, grape-growing regions will become less suitable for viticulture in California and shift into western North America where suitability is expected to increase by over 200 percent. The shift will potentially replace native habitats with the nonnative species of wine grapes.

"Plants in the wetland clean and re-oxygenate the water. The microbes living on the roots of the plants do 99 percent of the cleaning. You can say the microbes scrub the water. The hollow stems of the papyrus and other plants pump air into the water each time they sway to the motion of the wind."

"All the water used on this property ends up in those ponds?" I know the answer, but I need to hear it again aloud.

"Yeah," he says with a playful smugness. "Every drop we pump from the well is used twice. First, for cleaning and bottling in the winery, and second, to irrigate the vines. Most years that's enough water to do all of our irrigation. Some years we even have more water than we need, but this year we will need every drop."

"Is your well replenished with the rain?"

"Not even close. When we started in the '80s, we could pump 350 gallons a minute. Now it's less than sixty. The old thinking was, during every winter the aquifers will refill, but that's not the case. The groundwater, what I call our 'antique' water because it took hundreds of thousands of years to store, has been drawn down in less than fifty years."

"What about the surrounding vineyards? Do they use groundwater to irrigate and bottle the wine?"

"Most wineries in this area get their water exclusively from wells. Some growers get their water from the Russian River, but by far the vineyards use groundwater."

Twenty percent of all groundwater withdrawals in the US are in California, used predominately for irrigation.[245] In 2015, the California state legislature passed a law requiring permits to pump water. The new law will go into effect in 2040. Until then, any individual can build a well and pump unlimited amounts of water. When wells dry up, home-

245. Jay Feriglietti and Sasha Richley, "Sucking California Dry," *LA Times*, September 2013. One-third of the statewide supply is groundwater, higher during drought years.

owners, farms, and small towns are faced with two options: spend thousands of dollars for a deeper well or import costly water in tankers.[246]

"How deep are wells drilled on vineyards in this area?" I ask.

"The average is about 1,000 feet. Our well is 350 feet deep."

"Has lowered groundwater levels affected this property?"

"You see the creek over there?" He points to an area beyond the dirt road. It is difficult to see signs of a creek. "You can't see it because it has no flow. The groundwater no longer feeds the creek. At one time, the creek was the most prolific salmon creek in Northern California. The Indians settled on this land, mined obsidian in these hills, and could take salmon out of the creek by hand. The last salmon I saw in this creek was in 1981."

Mike and I slip back into the seats of the tram. "Next I'm going to take you to the insectary, where our domestic waste goes."

"Like from the toilets?" I say, dumbfounded.

"Yeah." He smiles, enjoying my reaction. "The waste from the toilet is piped to collect right under the insectary." Within minutes, we arrive. To any observer it is an herb and vegetable garden lined with fruit trees.

"One of the things we did when we started practicing biodynamics twenty years ago was hire an entomologist to study the different diseases and pests we have on this property. The standard practice is that the entomologist calls a chemical salesman, and they put a spray program together for you. What we did instead is put the entomologist in touch with a horticulturist. Together they designed this garden to attract beneficial insects."

"What bugs are beneficial?"

"Bees, lace bugs, spider mites, lady bugs. These are all insects that eat the bad bugs on our property like white flies, mites, and wasps. After we built this first insectary, we invited graduate students from UC Berkeley to study the migration patterns. With that information, we built

---

246. "Drought Forces Texas Town to Truck in Water," *CBS News*, January 31, 2012.

other insectaries. The insects travel between each creating highways. Over time, we developed this self-regulatory system between predator and prey."

"How well does this system work to eliminate pests?"

"It works 100 percent. I won't say it's bulletproof, but it works."

We walk further into the insectary. Poppies, grasses, lavenders, sages, and spiny ocotillos line the gravel path crunching under our shoes. We stop to pick ripe cherries dangling from a tree like earrings. We snack on a handful as we walk toward the raised beds of yarrow, chamomile, and valerian.

"The herbs we grow in our garden are used in the biodynamic teas. We dry and grind the herbs in tea machines and apply teas on the soil or mix them into the compost."

"What purpose do the teas serve?"

"They're medicines. They aid in deeper and wider root growth to help the grape vines grow with less water and other inputs."

"How?"

"Biodynamics acknowledges farming is a violent practice. You rip open the land, drive over it, and create oxidation. You need to have a healing practice build the immune system of the property."

His words resonate. I think of the farms near my home 300 miles away. Every few months the crop land is tilled, sprayed with chemicals, and often covered with white plastic like bandages.

"Do you need to apply the biodynamic medicine at a specific time?" I ask.

"Yes, we work from a calendar based on the movement of the sun and moon. Those movements are interpreted through the four elements: earth, water, air, and fire."

"It explains the four elements design on your wine logo," I say. He smiles in acknowledgment.

"In biodynamics we work within the natural rhythms of nature. When a plant is outside its rhythm, it is open to disease. Modern agriculture depends on inputs of water, chemicals, and fertilizers because they operate outside of the natural rhythms of nature."

We get back inside tram.

"You haven't seen one thing today that didn't happen for the first ten thousand years of agriculture. We're using old ideas and doing them more efficiently because we have the technology. The laws of nature remain the same now as they did thousands of years ago."

We arrive in front of the Craftsman-style tasting room.

"The whole purpose of all this is to create a liquid portrait of everything that happened in the year. If the plant has been under stress, fed chemicals, or watered too often, its portrait is shallow." He leaves me with a bottle of Cabernet Sauvignon before he drives away.

Inside the tasting room, I weave between thirsty people. I find a spot at the long dark wood counter. The man behind the counter pours me a few ounces of wine to taste. I hold the wine in my mouth. The flavor is extraordinary. It is a liquid portrait of deep root systems, healthy soil, and less water.

CHAPTER 14

Tequila & Water

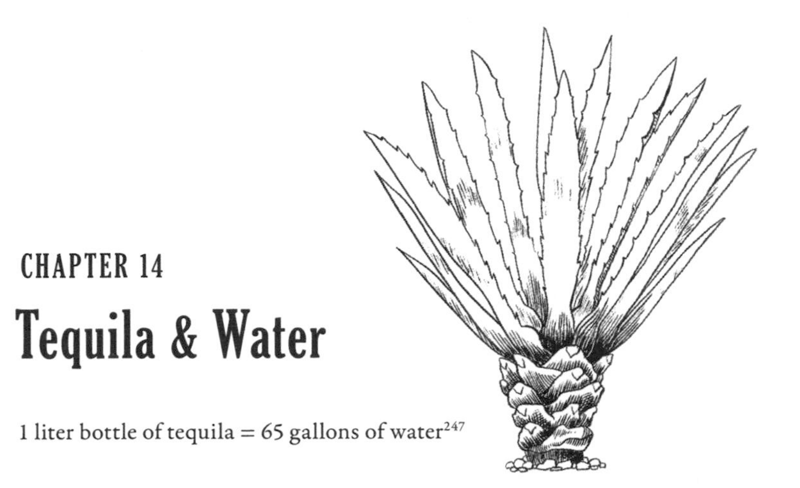

1 liter bottle of tequila = 65 gallons of water[247]

***BLANCO* TEQUILA IS** the color of water, too young to absorb the color of oak. It's the favored choice for margaritas, the most popular tequila drink. The US imports two-thirds of all tequila produced. Annually Americans sip, gulp, and mix 151 million liters of tequila, with a water footprint of nearly 10 billion gallons, enough to fill 17,845 Olympic-size pools.[248]

I swirl the clear liquid in my shot glass. Absent are wedges of lime and shakers of salt used to soften the sharp burn of tequila. Tequila Alquimia—the Spanish word for alchemy—is made to sip. Dr. Adolfo Murillo, owner of Tequila Alquimia, hands me a second taster.[249]

"Notice the color of the gold *añejo*," directs Adolfo. "Its color comes from oak barrels. We took minerals deep in the earth, rainwater from the sky, and energy from the sun and created liquid gold."

Gold medals prominently displayed in glass cases decorate the dining room in Adolfo's Oxnard, California, home. His tequilas *blanco*, *reposado*, *añejo*, and extra *añejo*, won forty international gold medals.

---

247. Kostigen, *The Green Blue Book*.
248. "Información Básica De La Industria Tequilera: Actualización al 11 de Enero, 2016," National Chamber of Tequila Industry, December 31, 2015: 1–11, http://www.tequileros.org/stuff/file_estadistica/1452616307.pdf.
249. Dr. Adolfo Murillo in discussion with the author, May 2012.

"Do judges know your tequila is organic?"

"No, it's a blind taste. Otherwise, it would be a small competition. There are only four certified USDA organic, out of 1,150 brands," Adolfo says. His thick, black mustache lifts with his smile.

"Do you think organic agave improves the flavor of your tequila?"

"My grandfather taught me if you treat the earth well, it will treat you well. So yes, how we grow the plants improves the flavor of the tequila."

He shows me photographs of his agave ranch in Agua Negra, Jalisco, one of five states that can cultivate tequila according to Mexican laws. The 125-acre ranch is adjacent to land that once belonged to Adolfo's grandfather. Dozens of photographs show the spiny blue agave plants growing in obedient straight lines. The strong, sharp spines reach for the sky in a sun salutation. Photos of cows, foraging between the tight rows of blue agave, enter the screen.

"The cattle are weed control," Adolfo says. "They increase the microbiological material of the soil with the manure they leave behind."

"Don't the cattle damage the agave plants?"

"No, they avoid the spines. I chose the Limousine cattle, originally from France, because of their superior foraging. The cattle help remove the *quiotes* every spring."

"What are *quiotes*?"

He leads me out through the sliding glass door near the kitchen and points upward. Blue agave border the patio of his home. My vision travels up along a thick stalk bursting from the center of one plant. Its top reaches the eaves of the second story. Clusters of corral-like flowers sprout from branches, the *quiote*.

"When you grow agave for tequila, you want the juice concentrated in the *piña* or core. *Quiotes*," he motions to the flower high above us, "extract significant juice from the plant, so we'd spend hours removing them by hand every spring. The cows began eating the flowers straight from the plant as soon as they figured out how sweet they taste. They do the work for us."

"Do other agave farms use cattle?"

"No, but the word has gotten out about our cows who eat *quiotes*. We considered renting them out, but we'd prefer that our cows eat only organic plants."

"How long does agave grow?" Standing beside one plant I touch the point of its leaf with the tip of my finger.

"Agaves grow for six to ten years. It depends on the timing of the harvest. The length of the growing season makes organic even more important. Most conventionally grown crops like lettuce or celery are cultivated in a single season. But the exposure to pesticides for agave spans years."

Agave farms depend on the steady application of chemicals to kill weeds and eradicate pests like the *picudo* bug or weevil. The glossy black insects with horn-shaped snouts feast on the sweet sap inside the leaves. Once inside the cavity of the plant, the *picudo* leaves its larvae behind, making the plant useless for distillation.

"Chemical fertilizers leave a residue of salts and heavy metals that collect in the soil after each use," Adolfo says. "Eventually, the land becomes less productive, causing the grower to use even more fertilizers. You end up with sterile soil that cannot sustain life."

Adolfo works to reverse the trend toward sterile land in Mexico. On his frequent trips to his ranch, he regularly mentors Mexican farmers on transitioning to organic farming.

"Why are your plants resistant to pests without chemicals?"

"When you use pesticides, the plant relies on the chemical instead of itself. Our plants build their own defenses."

Plants, unlike animals, have no immune system. The plant equivalent is a combination of structural, chemical, and protein-based defenses against pathogens. Nutrient imbalances compromise the plant's innate defense mechanisms and lower pest resistance, inviting the need to use chemicals to protect susceptible crops.

"The distillation process concentrates the chemicals absorbed by the plant over a decade. I believe it's why tequila's earned the reputation for terrible hangovers."

"I don't need to worry about a hangover?" I take a sip of the tequila from the shot glass I carried outside.

"No, but just like any alcohol, we all have our limits." I bring down the glass from my lips, unwilling to test mine.

We return to the photos on the laptop. The town of Agua Negra receives little rainfall. Close-ups of the ground reveal brittle sandstone. The water for irrigation comes primarily from underground. Eighty percent of large distilleries purchase agave from contract farmers.[250] Once the aquifer runs dry, leased land is abandoned, leaving limited water for small farms of the region.

Adolfo's agave is *dry* farmed, using no irrigation after the plant is established.

"How can you dry farm?"

"During the rainy season, we fence the cattle out of the agave to let the weeds grow. The weeds protect the topsoil and help store water. After the rainy season passes, we mow the weeds, leaving the root systems intact. We leave the mowed weeds on the ground, too. The decomposing plant material helps the soil absorb moisture for the plants in the dry months." Adolfo's farm collects millions of gallons of water under the parched rocks.

"My grandfather would invite the townspeople to use water from the spring on his land. I think it brought him a sense of pride to share water with his community."

---

250. Nagarajan S, "Agave Supply Crisis and Mitigation Strategies for Tequila Distillers," *Beverage Industry*, March 26, 2014, http://www.bevindustry.com/articles/87318-agave-supply-crisis-and-mitigation-strategies-for-tequila-distillers.

"Do you know what's happened to the spring?"

"The last I heard, it's nearly dry. I imagine the water is polluted with herbicides, pesticides, and fertilizers." His tone softens when speaking about his grandfather's land.

A picture of his two daughters holding machetes appears on the screen. "My daughters have become experts at using a machete," laughs Adolfo. Tequila is harvested by slicing off the leaves with machetes to expose the torso of the agave plant, called the *piña* (named so because it resembles an overgrown pineapple). Mules carry the ripe *piñas*, weighing between 80–200 pounds—more than three times the average weight of plants from surrounding farms. The sugar content, or Brix, of the *piña* adds to the complexity of flavor. Adolfo's Brix is more than double the average.

The images move from the farm to a tequila distillery located on a river. "Ancient alchemists invented distillation," Adolfo tells me.

Agave is cooked until it's soft and tastes like sweet potato. Next, it is shredded to release the juice from the plant fibers. Natural yeast eats the sugars and digests them, creating alcohol in fermentation tanks twice Adolfo's height.

"The fermentation will take seven to ten days when you let it follow its natural course, as we do. Many tequila companies prefer the faster method of three days, using supercharged yeast that's essentially chemical fertilizer." The heavy metals and salt present in the supercharged yeast is concentrated during distillation.

"Tequila production leaves behind *vinaza*, a liquid that holds high concentrations of chemicals, heavy metals, salt, and nitrogen."

What happens to the *vinaza*?" I ask, afraid of the answer.

"The common practice of *vinaza* disposal is to pour it untreated into rivers." We look at photos posted on the Internet of rivers tainted with tequila's byproduct. The river water is the color of rust. The Mexican government discourages the practice of dumping untreated *vinazas* by imposing fines. Most distilleries opt to pay the fines rather than building costly treatment plants. Every one-liter bottle of tequila generates ten liters of *vinazas*.

Adolfo devised a solution for *vinaza* disposal. "On the land behind the distillery, we turn the vinaza into compost. We pour *vinaza* over a layer of clay and *piña* fiber." He shows me a picture of weeds and flowers growing out of a mound of soil. "With a little bit of effort, *vinaza* can support life instead of stripping the rivers of Mexico of their ability to sustain life."

One last sip of tequila remains. I raise my glass, and Adolfo joins in. "To Tequila Alquimia! Thank you for preserving fresh water supplies and protecting rivers." Our glasses chime in agreement.

Alquimia-rita

Measurements for 2 margaritas provided

The following recipe is the best margarita you will ever taste. After you try a margarita with fresh juice it's hard to go back to margarita mix made with high fructose corn syrup, food coloring, and cellulose gum (extracted from wood pulp and cotton cellulose).

Support one of the handful of organic tequila makers and email your favorite brand asking how they dispose of their *vinaza*. Let's protect rivers in Mexico one drink at a time. Salud!

Ingredients

- 2 parts Alquimia *Blanco* or other certified organic tequila (3 ounces)
- 2 parts organic fresh lime juice (3 ounces)
- 1 part organic orange juice (1.5 ounces)
- 1 part organic agave sweetener (1.5 ounces)

Directions

1. Add ingredients in a shaker with ice.
2. Shake till very cold.
3. Serve over ice.

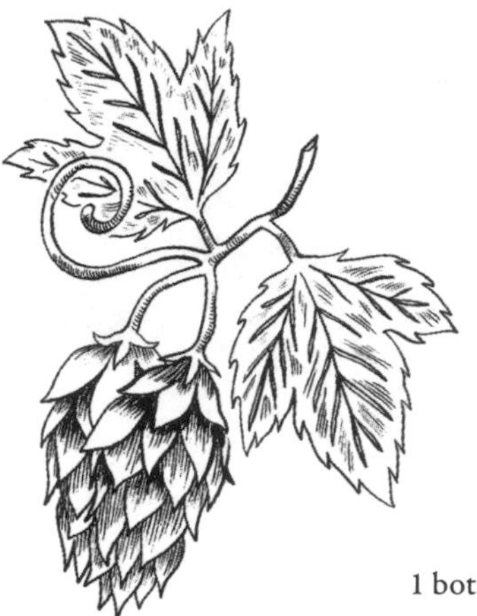

CHAPTER 15

Beer & Water

1 bottle of beer = 29.6 gallons of water

1 six-pack of beer = 178 gallons of water[251]

SAVE WATER. DRINK BEER. If only it were so easy. With a virtual water footprint of nearly thirty gallons per glass, America's adult beverage of choice is a strain on water systems and wastewater treatment facilities. But can we save water *and* drink beer? I took my question to Helen and Mike Cameron, owners of Greenstar Brewery, the first certified organic brewery in Illinois.

I meet with Helen and Mike in their North Chicago restaurant, Uncommon Ground. The husband and wife team remind me of beer glasses; Mike, a tall Pilsner glass for lagers, and Helen, a curved tulip glass reserved for strong or dark ales.[252] They guide me away from the vibrant chatter of customers enjoying Saturday morning brunch to an empty adjoining dining room.

We take our seats around the table. Martin, the brewmaster, joins us with a flight of four tasters each containing different shades of amber. "People are awakening to what's in their food, but they don't extrapolate into what they're drinking," says Helen.

251. Kostigen, *The Green Blue Book*.

252. Helen Cameron and Mike Cameron in discussion with the author, July 2016.

I reach for the first taster of Spaceship Pale Ale. Drinking beer before breakfast is a first for me.

"Breakfast of champions," I say, taking my first sip.

"Beer is food," says Martin. His smile appears behind his scruffy beard.

"I think of beer as soup," says Helen, gesturing for me to take another sip. "It can be a healthful thing. Fermented foods like beer are good for digestion." I finish the first taster of tasty beer soup.

Fermentation dates back to 7000 BC. Bacteria or yeast, fed by sugar in the food, is converted to alcohol or lactic acid during fermentation. Eating or drinking fermented foods promotes microbial balance in the gut, the largest component of our immune system, making it easier for the body to digest and absorb nutrients. A healthy gastrointestinal tract reduces inflammation linked to a range of health disorders from allergies to autoimmune diseases.[253]

The fermentation process can be likened to microorganisms in the soil. Sugar in roots and plant material feeds microorganisms. A thriving microbial community in the ground increases the availability of nutrients to a plant and heightens the plant's resistance to disease and pests.[254]

"I'm convinced that organic beer is healthier than conventionally brewed beer," says Mike. "During a party to celebrate the twenty-fifth anniversary of Uncommon Ground, a few of my gluten-intolerant friends drank three pints, figuring they would suffer the consequences

---

253. I reviewed several websites and studies on the fermented foods. I found the following the most helpful: "Discover the Digestive Benefits of Fermented Food," Tufts University Gerald J. and Dorothy R. Friedman School of Nutrition Science and Policy, February 2014, http://www.nutritionletter.tufts.edu/issues/10_2/current-articles/Discover-the-Digestive-Benefits-of-Fermented-Foods_1383-1.html. Katie Klein, "Spontaneous fermentation: the role of microorganisms in beer," Ecological Society of America, September 10, 2010, http://www.esa.org/esablog/research/spontaneous-fermentation-the-role-of-microorganisms-in-beer.

254. Elaine Ingham, Andrew R. Moldenke and Clive A. Edwards, "Soil Biology," USDA Natural Resources Conservation Service, https://www.nrcs.usda.gov/wps/portal/nrcs/main/soils/health/biology.

later. Three out of four reported they felt no symptoms. It got me wondering if the real reason for gluten issues is not just the wheat crop but the chemicals applied to the grain."

"Why is it suddenly people are unable to digest gluten?" Helen wonders aloud. "What has changed from the time we were kids? I think there is something about the chemicals sprayed on the wheat that's causing problems for human health. While there is no GMO wheat on the market, Roundup is sprayed on wheat at the end of its growth cycle because it's a desiccant and makes it easier to harvest the grain. I don't know if there is a connection between this practice and gluten problems, but what I can say is I don't want those chemicals in my food or drink stream."

"In Germany, beer is brewed with malt, water, hops, and yeast," says Martin. "No chemical additives are allowed in brewing. It's the law, and it's been the law for 500 years. But an environmental group found a surprisingly large number of beers with Roundup in the finished beer. Although German brewers only use malt, water, hops, and yeast, it's not organic. Organic is not the law."

The German beer purity law regulates the ingredients of Europe's largest beer producer. The 500-year-old law does not monitor contamination of the mandated ingredients. A 2016 study found traces of glyphosate, the leading ingredient in Roundup Ready, in fourteen of Germany's most popular beers. The presence of the herbicide in beer was up to 300 times higher than the allowable limit in water.[255]

"Why aren't there more certified organic breweries, both large and small?" I ask them while I continue my private beer tasting. Organic

---

255. Caroline Copley, "German Beer Purity in Question after Environment Group Finds Weed-killer Traces," *Reuters*, February 25, 2016, http://www.reuters.com/article/us-germany-beer-idUSKCN0VY222. Traces of the herbicide were between 0.46 micrograms to 29.74 micrograms per liter. The limit for drinking water is 0.1 microgram.

beer sales grew 922 percent in a little over a decade. Despite the surge, organic beer represents less than 1 percent of all beer sales in the US.[256]

"The top myths I've heard from other breweries are: organic beer is too expensive, organic ingredients are hard to find, and consistent quality is hard to achieve," says Martin.

"We've disproved all those myths," says Helen.

"For example," says Martin, "when others learn I brew organic beer the first reaction is, 'organic beer must be so expensive.' The answer is no. Organic ingredients are a bit more expensive, but as far as cost per pint it does not make a noticeable difference."

"We're talking pennies," says Mike. "Organic certification does cost money, but it's not going to hurt your bottom line in a brewery."

"What about consistency?" I ask.

"Consistency was an issue in the past," Martin tells me, who started, like so many brewmasters, as a home brewer, then worked for a large German brewery before Greenstar.

"A decade ago, farmers didn't know how to grow quality hops and barley. Now, more people are getting into the growing of organic ingredients," says Mike. "And the availability of quality organic products has grown."

"To be blunt, consistency is more of a brewing issue. Every single brewer, whether you are working with organic ingredients or not, has the challenge of making a consistent product. Because you're working with agricultural ingredients that vary every season because of weather shifts, your recipe can never be 'the recipe.' Slight modifications are required if you want the beer to taste the same every single time," Martin tells me.

"Was it difficult locating organic ingredients?" I ask.

---

256. "National Beer Sales & Production Data—Brewers Association," Brewers Association, https://www.brewersassociation.org/statistics/national-beer-sales-production-data.

Helen answers, "When we brought Martin to work with us, we told him, 'Here's the challenge, you must certify the brewery organic. Can you find enough sources?'"

"It wasn't nearly as hard to locate ingredients as everyone first thought," remembers Martin. "I called this large corporate beer supplier for organic ingredients, and he told me the only people who are crazy enough to brew organic beer in your location are the gluten-free brewers. So in honor of his erroneous judgment, we called our first beer Certifiable American Pale Ale," Martin points out the APA in my beer flight.

"Do you purchase from local farms?" I ask.

"We buy from farms here in Illinois, Michigan, and Wisconsin," answers Martin.

"Our hops are purchased from a Midwest cooperative of a dozen organic farmers. They recently came to the brewery for a tour and tasting. It was gratifying when they told us as their biggest customer we make it possible for them to grow organic hops," says Mike.

"We're changing the way people view organic beer. You don't need to choose between organic beer or good beer. Organic beer is both," says Helen. "The more we build a local following, the more we can support local farmers and get them to succeed because we're supporting those crops."

I raise my morning beer for a toast; they join me with their glasses of water, beer's essential ingredient.

Mike leaves to tend to the restaurant. Helen and I follow Martin into the brewery located through a door.

~

Tall stainless steel tanks line the walls of unfinished wood and exposed brick. The air swirls with the sweet and bitter scents of hops and malt. We stand in front of the first shiny silver tank. "The brewing process begins with malt," says Martin. "Malt is crushed and mixed with water, called a mash to extract sugars from the grain. At this stage, some conventional brewers add chemical additives for pH and to regulate the temperature. Organic brewers can't add *any* chemicals to beer, nor would I want to."

"What do you do to check the pH and the temperature?"

"I follow the German technique. Instead of chemicals, I use an acidified type of malt that naturally lowers the pH. Or, I add a small amount of a lactobacillus, considered a friendly bacterium that eats sugars."

"Have you always brewed organic?"

"I didn't set out to be an organic brewer. I just questioned the need for additives. I learned early on that all you need to make good beer is to pay attention to the process and use quality ingredients," says Martin.

"Are home brewers using chemical additives too?"

"The same chemicals available to brewers are available to home brewers in small packets. Home brewers are taught to include additives, both plant- or animal-derived like Irish moss and isinglass, and chemically derived additives like silicone. Companies that manufacture additives are smart to market to home brewers, because that's the training ground for many commercial brewers. They're essentially raising the next generation of chemically dependent beer makers," says Martin.

New labeling rules issued by the Food and Drug Administration (FDA) requires beer labels to list nutritional breakdowns, fluid ounces, alcohol content, and ingredients. Indirect food additives, such as dimethylpolysiloxane, a silicone, or Irish moss, a carrageenan, included during the beer-making process do not need to be listed.

"After the mash, you have leftover grain. The spent grain contains sugar, protein, and nutrients. We give most of our spent grains to a local farmer for her animals. The rest Helen uses in her recipes," says Martin.

"You can use the spent grain when it's wet, or you can slowly oven-dry and pulverize it, turning it into flour," says Helen. "We serve spent grain burgers in the restaurant. In the past we've served pizza made from spent grain. We're always experimenting with new recipes."

"What typically happens to spent grain in American breweries?"

"Some breweries throw the stuff out in the dumpster," Martin tells me. "But there is a growing trend for breweries both big and small to sell or give it away."

We step over to an identical tank. "Boiling is the next step. Hops get added and additional chemicals. Not by me of course," Martin is quick to add.

"Let me guess: the chemical additive keeps the liquid from boiling over," I say partly in jest.

"How did you know?" he asks. "The sweet liquid can boil over and needs to be monitored closely. Or, as you guessed, you can add a chemical additive. It's completely possible to brew good beer without adding all this extra stuff. Organic beer is about getting back to the basics of brewing."

We step to the final tank. "Liquid is pumped around in a whirlpool to separate hop matter and protein sediment from the clean wort, the ground malt, and grain before fermentation. Breweries use a lot of water during this step. Our system is set up to return the water to the tank where it is reused for subsequent batches," says Martin.

"How much water do you use?"

"Most breweries have around a 4:1 ratio of water to beer. I've gotten our water use down to 3:1 just by using this closed-loop system."

Innovations to save water at the brewery are important. This is especially true when breweries are tapped to water sources in short supply. But even in regions where the water supply is abundant, breweries with high water use stress local wastewater treatment facilities. According to a manual written by the Brewers Association, 2 liters of beer generates between 4–17.4 liters of wastewater.[257] Most breweries discharge 70 per-

257. "Water and Wastewater: Treatment/Volume Reduction Manual," Brewers Association: 17, https://www.brewersassociation.org/attachments/0001/1517/Sustainability_-_Water_Wastewater.pdf.

cent of their wastewater to the sewer systems, and few breweries have dedicated onsite wastewater treatment system to treat the wastewater, as recommended by the Brewers Association. This effluent water contains high levels of nitrogen and phosphorus, two leading causes of oxygen depletion in surface water.

While water conservation at the brewery is necessary, about 99.7 percent of the water footprint to produce a twelve-ounce bottle of beer flows to the field to grow hops, barley, and malt. The water footprint for a bottle of beer is higher when recipes include corn and rice, water-intensive crops. For a brewery to save water, the brewer must look to the fields growing crops, and support farmers growing crops with less *blue* water for irrigation and who use few to no chemicals that leech into waterways. When a brewer's water-conservation plan extends beyond the brewery and onto the fields, he is protecting clean water, beer's most essential ingredient.

Martin points to the fermentation tank. "The wort goes in here, with yeast and—" He pauses.

"More additives?" I guess.

"Most brewers will include additives to clarify and to speed up the fining process."

An array of additives is available to clarify beer, referred to as fining. Some include chitosan (skeleton of shellfish), kieselsol (colloidal silica), isinglass (fish bladder), and Irish moss (carrageenan). Compelling evidence links carrageenan, a common thickening ingredient in conventional and certified organic dairy and meat, to inflammation. Many organic food brands have voluntarily removed carrageenan from food in response to consumer concern.[258]

---

258. Sumit Bhattacharyya, Leo Feferman, and Joanne K. Tobacman, "Carrageenan Inhibits Insulin Signaling through GRB10-mediated Decrease in Tyr(P)-IRS1 and through Inflammation-induced Increase in Ser(P)307-IRS1," *The Journal of Biological Chemistry*, March 15, 2015, http://www.jbc.org/content/290/17/10764. Removing the thickening agent made from red seaweed from the list of approved organic ingredients is under review by the National Organic Standards Board (NOSB).

~

"After fermentation, it's typical for breweries to filter their beer," says Martin.

"We made a conscious decision not to filter," says Helen. "When you remove the yeast you remove vitamins and proteins."

"Why filter?"

"Filtering is entirely cosmetic. Let me show you what I mean," Martin looks over at my empty taster glass. "Follow me." We follow him back to the bustling dining room. Helen and I pull up a seat at the bar.

"This is not our beer, it's a guest tap." Martin holds a glass in front of us to inspect the contents. "If you can see through the liquid, it's filtered."

"Filtered beer removes the yeast. It's like the difference between apple cider and apple juice," explains Helen. "You don't see through apple cider because there are tiny particles in suspension."

Martin holds up the second glass of Greenstar's IPA. The gold liquid is opaque. "Unfiltered beer is cloudy."

Martin hands me a taster of Greenstar Moonless Midnight Imperial Stout, the last beer to sample before I sink my teeth into the scrumptious food served at Uncommon Ground. Chocolate, nutmeg, and vanilla with hints of pine from the hops brighten my palette. I resist the urge to drink the entire taster in one gulp. This beer speaks my language.

"Which is your favorite beer?"

Helen answers, "Blackcurrant Kölsch. It's an homage to my mother. She was from Cologne, Germany, and drank blackcurrant nectar when she was pregnant with me. We grow the blackcurrants on our rooftop farm." The first certified organic rooftop farm in the country is the next stop on the tour.

~

Every square inch of usable rooftop space is cultivated. Raised boxes of chard with magenta veins and stems are paired with flowering heirloom tomatoes climbing on trellises. Sturdy kale leaves form a backdrop to lacy white petals of coriander. Edible flowers of nasturtiums, pansies, and violas add splashes of orange, yellow, and purple to the sea of green plants. Solar panels line one corner, beehives the other.

"How much do you grow on this rooftop?" I ask Helen.

"Conventional farmers are ecstatic to grow two pounds per square foot. Last year, we grew 15 thousand pounds on 800 square feet, 3.71 pounds per square foot. We use 100 percent of what we grow in our food and beer."

Plants are grown in raised beds called EarthBoxes. The box is designed to lower evaporation from the top and retain the nutrients.

Hops grow along the perimeter of the rooftop. "We use it in our beer," says Helen. I reach to touch the dangling hops resembling young pine cones as green as sprouted grass.

"Our mission is to relocalize food systems," says Helen. "We have great water resources and soil in the Midwest, yet all we're producing is GMO corn. Everything we grow here in Illinois is shipped out of the state, forcing people to purchase food from everywhere else. It's absurd."

The amber and clear lights strung across this urban farm sway with the errant summer Chicago breeze.

"All big cities can grow a measure of their food. We're proving it can be done."

Michael's Organic Dark Ale Two-Bean Chili with Beef or Tempeh

Makes 8 large servings

20 minutes to prepare

100 minutes to cook

On Halloween, family and friends join us to eat bowls of my husband Michael's chili and to help distribute candy to more than one thousand trick-or-treaters who come to our front door. It's become a tradition. A new tradition is the addition of organic porter in our chili to accompany the glasses of organic beer soup and a pot of tempeh chili. Tempeh is a nutritious fermented soy. It makes an exceptional alternative to meat due to its nutty texture and its easy adherence to spices.

Ingredients

2 pounds organic rotationally grazed, pasture-raised ground beef[259] or organic soy or 2 pounds organic tempeh (fermented soybeans)

1 tablespoon organic canola oil (needed if cooking tempeh)

2 cups organic onion, chopped (1 medium onion)

2 tablespoons organic chili powder

1 tablespoon salt

1 tablespoon organic garlic powder

1½ teaspoons organic paprika

259. See "Chapter 10: Meat & Water."

1 teaspoon dried organic thyme
1 teaspoon ground black pepper
½ teaspoon organic cayenne pepper
¼ teaspoon organic cumin
2 cups water
½ cup organic all-purpose flour (preferably dry farmed)[260]
2 cups cooked organic black beans with liquid or 1 (15 ounce) can of organic black beans with the liquid
2 cups cooked organic kidney beans with liquid or 1 (15 ounce) can organic kidney beans with the liquid*
1 (15 ounce) can organic diced tomatoes
1 (12 ounce) bottle organic dark ale (porter or stout)

GARNISHES

2 cups organic cheddar cheese (Choose dairy from farms practicing rotation grazing)[261]
½ cup organic sour cream (see note on dairy)
½ cup organic green onions, chopped

Directions

FOR GROUND BEEF:

1. Brown ground beef in a large saucepan or Dutch oven. Drain excess fat. Add chopped onion and spices to the meat and sauté for an additional 5 minutes.
2. Continue to step 3 below.

FOR TEMPEH:

1. Heat canola oil in large saucepan or Dutch oven.

---

260. See "Chapter 1: Wheat & Water." for a discussion on dry farming.
261. See "Chapter 9: Dairy & Water" or "Chapter 10: Meat & Water" for further discussion on the importance of supporting intensive managed rotationally grazed systems.

2. Crumple tempeh and add to the skillet and sauté for 5–8 minutes. Mix in all spices and chopped onion. Cook for an additional 5 minutes.
3. Combine flour with water in a bowl and add to saucepan of ground beef or tempeh.
4. Add tomatoes and beer and bring chili to a simmer. Simmer uncovered for 1.5 hours, stirring occasionally.
5. Garnish with cheese, sour cream, and green onions.

Greenstar Spent Grain Burgers

Makes 8 burger patties or 16 sliders

30 minutes to prepare

30 minutes to cook

Ingredients

¼ cup uncooked organic quinoa
½ cup water
pinch of salt
1 tablespoon olive oil
1 medium organic carrot, shredded
1 medium organic onion, finely diced
1 organic celery stalk, chopped fine
2 cups organic mushrooms, chopped
4 small organic garlic cloves, minced
1 cup wet barley spent grain from a variety of beer with low bitterness*
2 organic pasture-raised eggs[262]
¾ teaspoon salt
½ cup panko plus more if needed
2 tablespoons unseasoned organic tomato sauce
1 tablespoon local honey
1 tablespoon fresh organic orange juice
1 teaspoon organic dijon mustard

262. See "Chapter 7: Eggs & Water."

1 teaspoon organic smoked paprika

½ teaspoon organic balsamic vinegar

**Ask for spent grain from your favorite local microbrewery*

Directions

1. Pour uncooked quinoa in small saucepan with ½ cup water and salt and bring to a boil at medium-high heat. Lower heat, cover pot, and simmer for around 15 minutes until all water is absorbed. Let stand covered for a few minutes, then fluff with a fork and let cool.
2. Heat olive oil in sauté pan and add onions, garlic, celery, mushrooms, and carrots and allow the liquid to evaporate and veggies to brown slightly. Remove from heat and set aside.
3. Mix tomato sauce, honey, orange juice mustard, paprika, and vinegar in a large bowl.
4. Add quinoa, veggies, barley spent grain, salt, eggs, panko, and sauce into bowl. Mix well until all ingredients are well distributed and cohesive. Add more panko if mix is too wet.
5. Hand-form patties, 1 tablespoon for sliders or 2 tablespoons for larger patties and place on parchment paper.
6. Heat olive oil in a skillet or on a griddle. Cook the patties for 3–5 minutes undisturbed to allow a nice browned crust before very carefully flipping over and cooking another 2–3 minutes to brown other side.
7. Serve on toasted buns with your favorite flavors of the season.

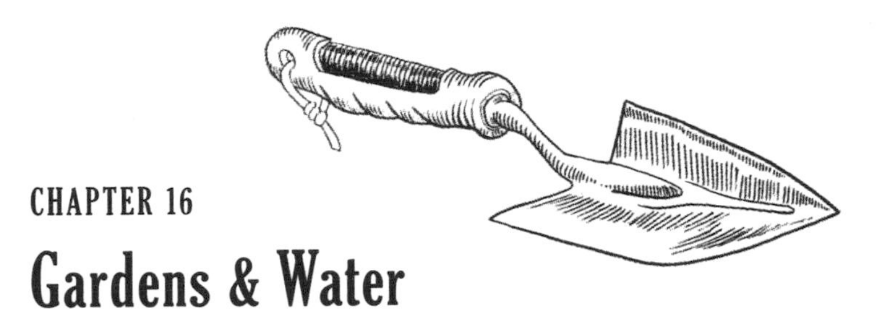

CHAPTER 16

Gardens & Water

1 sprinkler nozzle running for 30 minutes = 480 gallons of water

1 garden hose running for 30 minutes = 510 gallons of water[263]

IN THE UNITED States, the amount of paved land such as roads, driveways, and parking lots total an area larger than the state of Ohio. The rain glides across instead of through these surfaces, taking with it surface pollutants. The difference in the amount of run-off between paved and unpaved surfaces is tremendous. In woodland areas, 95 percent of the water is absorbed by the soil. In urbanized areas where large swaths of exposed land are paved, absorption decreases to 50 percent.[264] Water runs off these impervious surfaces fast, warm, and polluted.[265]

"About one hundred gardens harvest rain in NYC. Tanks collect around 1.1 million gallons a year," says Lenny Librizzi, Director of Green Infrastructure for the nonprofit GrowNYC.

"That's impressive."

"It is, but New Yorkers use 1.2 billion gallons of water *each day.* A million gallons is a drop in the bucket. But in NYC, rainwater harvest-

263. For these totals I used the data provided by the Washington Suburban Sanitary Commission, found online at http://www.wsscwater.com/home/jsp/content/water-usagechart.faces.

264. Lance Frazer, "Paving Paradise: The Peril of Impervious Surfaces," Environmental Health Perspectives 113, no. 7 (July 2005): A456-A462, https://www.ncbi.nlm.nih.gov/pmc/articles/PMC1257665/.

265. Ibid.

ing serves a dual purpose. It saves water and reduces pollution by diverting water from the combined sewer system."

"Combined sewer system?" I ask him to explain while we make our way along the bustling Manhattan sidewalk toward the GrowNYC work van parked five blocks away.

"Our sewer collects water from showers, the kitchen sink, garbage disposals, toilet flushes, etc. It's called 'sanitary waste.' These same pipes collect rainfall from storm water drains."

"What's wrong with this system?" I ask, not understanding how this leads to water pollution.

"The sewer can handle the sanitary waste just fine in dry weather, but overflows during a rain event. When the sewer overflows, untreated water is shunted directly into the bodies of water that surround us like the Hudson River, East River, and Jamaica Bay." An audible gasp escapes me. It seems inconceivable for sewage to gush untreated from the largest and most advanced metropolitan area in the country.

We arrive at the work van.

"How much rainfall overflows the system?" I ask Lenny as I move an assortment of garden tools from the passenger seat.

"It doesn't take much. Overflows can happen with as little as one-tenth to one-fourth of an inch of rain; twenty-seven billion gallons of untreated waste per year is dumped into the water bodies around NYC."

"Why doesn't the city modernize its combined sewage system or expand its wastewater treatment–holding capacity?"

"It's cost prohibitive to separate the storm and sanitary sewers. This is why storm water–management techniques like rainwater-harvesting systems are critical."

An estimated 772 US communities, representing 40 million Americans, have active combined sewer systems (CSS) with the majority located in the Northeast, Pacific Northwest, and the Great Lakes regions.[266] NYC is the largest metropolitan area with a CSS. In dry weather, the CSS channels raw human and industrial waste to a treatment plant, then discharges the treated water into adjoining waterways.[267] In wet weather, the sewer diverts the combined rainfall, snowmelt, bacteria, viruses from human waste, oil, grease, trash from streets, chemicals, and nutrients from croplands into bordering oceans, lakes, and every major river—untreated.

The EPA estimates Combined Sewer Overflows (CSOs) are to blame for 3,500–5,500 gastrointestinal illnesses each year in the Great Lakes area and coastal beaches. In 2000, the Clean Water Act was strengthened to reduce or eliminate CSS overflows. The volume of raw sewage dumped into US waters has decreased but more than 860 billion gallons continue to overflow annually.[268]

The doors of the van rattle as we drive over the Verrazano-Narrows Bridge toward Staten Island. New York Bay extends below. The indigo sky reflecting off the bay conceals the filth of untreated sewage dumped into the bay during every rainfall.

In Staten Island, we travel along the waterfront. Rusted debris washed up from Super Storm Sandy is still visible on the battered shore.

"In my part of the world, we receive too little rain. Do you find that you get too much rain here in the Northeast?" I ask.

"At GrowNYC and partner organizations, we have noticed the quality and quantity of the rainfall change in the last ten years. Rain events in the past were less severe, or at least the severe storms were much less frequent, of shorter duration, or contained less total rainfall."

---

266. "Keeping Raw Sewage and Contaminated Stormwater Out of the Public's Water," US EPA, 2011, http://www.epa.gov/region2/water/sewer-report-3-2011.pdf.
267. John Tibbetts, "Combined Sewer Systems: Down, Dirty, and Out of Date," *Environmental Health Perspectives* 113, no. 7 (July 2005): A464–467, http://www.ncbi.nlm.nih.gov/pmc/articles/PMC1257666.
268. "How Sewage Pollution Ends Up in Rivers," American Rivers, https://www.americanrivers.org/threats-solutions/clean-water/sewage-pollution.

The rain has a new implication for me now; when it rains, the sewer pours untreated wastewater. Which makes Lenny's charge to capture a portion of the ninety billion gallons of water that falls inside the borders of NYC that more critical.

We park in front of Lenny's house. The hundred-year-old Queen Anne is surrounded by a lush and colorful garden. Grass is absent.

Lenny is a curator of plants. He names the plants spilling over the walkway of sliced stone, joined with pervious sand. Every patch of earth is covered with the gold bursts of silphium, magenta of bee balm, and white flower cones of oakleaf hydrangea. His plants thrive on summer rain.

We walk through the house to the back door. His pack of small dogs barks at my heels. Only the miniature greyhound heeds Lenny's admonishments. The long, narrow backyard is host to a small ecosystem. Bantam chickens peck for insects near their henhouse; songbirds find respite on the crooked branches of maple trees overhead; bees buzz near the wooden hive.

My eyes fix on the back wall. "Are those tomatoes growing on the fence?" I walk toward it to get a closer look.

"Those are vertical planters. I plant the tomatoes in recycled bags typically used for construction projects for sand and gravel. I attach a few grommets to the bag and hang them on the wood fence. They work well for people who have limited growing spaces. I find that they work well for me because I'm low on sunny spots in this yard."

I reach to squeeze the hose snaked above the three rows of bags secured to the fence. It yields to my grip. "What kind of garden hose is this?"

"It is a soaker hose. It outputs a lot less water than a sprinkler or average garden hose. The water beads out of the surface like sweat on your skin."

"Do you prefer this over a drip system?"

"It works well in wet regions where we get freezing temperatures. Drip-system hoses expand and crack in freezing weather, so many of the drip systems in gardens around the city aren't working. You only need one crack in the header line and anything down river from it isn't getting any water." We follow the soaker hose to the side of the house, where it is attached to a spigot on the bottom of the rainwater tank.

"How many gallons of water does your tank hold?"

"Water-holding tanks come in different sizes. This tank holds 160 gallons. It collects water from one quarter of the roof. The bigger the roof, the larger the tank. With every inch of rain, roofs collect a half gallon of water per square foot. This roof collects 500 gallons of water with one inch of rain."

"What happens when you get more water than your tank can hold?"

"When the tank is full, the excess water is diverted into this rain garden planted with hostas." He points to the ground near the tank.

"What is a rain garden?"

"A rainwater-harvest system needs a surface to collect rainwater. It can be a roof, but in the case of a rain garden or swale, tree pit, or permeable surface, it's the ground. The rainwater is stored in the soil where microorganisms break down pollutants and recharge groundwater tables that feed surface waters."

Rain gardens and swales are shallow ditches, landscaped with drought- and drench-tolerant plants. A swale is long and narrow, but a rain garden can take any shape. Tree pits are carved openings in the sidewalk. Rainwater enters through the opening, collecting water around the tree and plants. Each is like a pocket in the ground, designed to pool and keep rainwater and snowmelt.

"The best-designed systems keep rain in the garden and out of the city sewer system, which keeps the soil moist longer and replenishes the water table." We walk through the diverse variety of the leafy hostas in the rain garden.

Cities around the US install rainwater catchment systems on publicly maintained properties. Twenty-three acres of swales and tree pits in NYC are estimated to prevent four million gallons of storm water from reaching the Combined Sewer Systems each year.[269] Since 2004, the city of Chicago began repaving its 1,900 miles of alleys with pervious paver or permeable asphalt under the Green Alley's program. These "green alleys" absorb up to 80 percent of rainwater, decrease persistent flooding of alleyways, recharge groundwater, and reduce storm water in sewers responsible for combined sewer overflows. The program now includes 3,775 miles of streets.[270]

"Are people in NYC incorporating rainwater-catchment strategies at home?"

"The city distributes fifty-gallon rain barrels to private homeowners, and I'm starting to see rain gardens or swales used in home gardens," says Lenny.

Though it is critical for publicly maintained properties to implement rainwater-harvesting strategies to curb water pollution and replenish shrinking water tables, the majority of the 2.3 billion acres of US land is privately owned, roughly 61 percent.[271]

~

269. Julia Chun-Heer, "Major Green Infrastructure Project Is Completed in New York," Surfrider Foundation, April 12, 2013, http://www.surfrider.org/coastal-blog/entry/major-green-infrastructure-project-is-completed-in-new-york.

270. "The Chicago Green Alley Handbook," City of Chicago, http://www.cityofchicago.org/dam/city/depts/cdot/Green_Alley_Handbook_2010.pdf. Janet L. Attarian, "Greener Alleys," Federal Highway Administration, Public Roads, May/June 2010, http://www.fhwa.dot.gov/publications/publicroads/10mayjun/05.cfm.

271. "State of the Land," Resources First Foundation, 2006, http://www.privatelandownernetwork.org/pdfs/StateoftheLand.pdf.

The fragrance of black licorice escapes the wispy leaves of fennel in the vegetable and herb garden. The ample patch is between the beehive and chicken coop.

"You don't use raised beds?"

"Raised beds are useful to mitigate contaminated soil, but level soil retains moisture best."

Water drains faster and evaporation occurs on the surface and four sides when soil is in pots or raised beds. Plants grown in the ground save water.

"How can home gardeners build their soil?"

"Collecting leaves and grass clippings. I keep it in one pile." I follow him to the compost behind the chicken coop. It is a discreet mound of decaying green waste.

"Gnats or flies aren't hovering. Do you separate your food scraps?"

"Yes, the kitchen scraps are kept in covered plastic tubs. An open pile of food waste is a feast for rodents, possums, raccoons, and flies."

"When do you mix your kitchen scraps in with the green yard waste?"

"When the food is no longer distinguishable, like when you can't tell what a tomato is or an apple core. At that point, I add them in with the clippings and leaves and turn the pile."

Compost is beneficial to water systems on many fronts. Compost, rich with micro-organisms, absorbs more water, a minimum of one half gallon per square foot of soil.[272]

Diverting kitchen scraps from landfills to compost piles reduces greenhouse gas in the atmosphere. The decomposition of food waste in landfills and wastewater treatment plants accounts for 20 percent of methane emissions. Methane is twenty-five times more harmful in

---

272. With every 1 percent increase of organic material (SOM) present in compost the water holding capacity increases by 20,000–25,000 gallons per acre of land. Using this measure, I divided 22,500 gallons of water, the average increase of water holding for 1 percent of SOM in the compost with 43,560, the number of square feet in an acre. For more discussion on this topic, see "Chapter 9: Dairy & Water."

terms of climate change than carbon dioxide.[273] Of the 40 percent of food thrown away in the US, only 3 percent is composted.[274]

"Cover crops is a technique organic farmers use to build nitrogen and one I use in this garden too," Lenny says.

The first time I learned of cover crops I was on a biodynamic wheat farm in Paso Robles, California. I've come to expect it on my farm visits, but it never occurred to me to grow cover crops in my home garden.

We stand at the border of his vegetable and herb patch. Comfrey, basil, and parsley are mixed in with rhubarb, lettuce, and beets. The black soaker hose curves around the plants, conspicuous against the scattered hay mulch.[275]

"When do you plant your cover crops?"

"Around Halloween, when I'm done with the crops for the year. For you, it would depend on when your season is over." He walks me through the steps.

"I scatter seeds of wheat, clover, or rye grass over my vegetable patch and turn the soil. Sometimes I put some compost down before I sow the seeds. If I need nitrogen fixers, I plant beans and clovers. I water the seeds enough to be sure the soil doesn't completely dry out until the crop cover is established. The plants will grow a little and might die back. Once the spring hits, they grow again, and you turn the crop cover into the soil."

---

273. "Methane Emissions," US EPA, September 9, 2013, https://web.archive.org/web/20170721221551/https://www.epa.gov/ghgemissions/overview-greenhouse-gases#methane; Gabriel Yvon-Durocher at al., "Methane fluxes show consistent temperature dependence across microbial to ecosystem scales. *Nature* 507, March 27, 2014: 488–491. Landfills are the third largest source of methane emission. The first largest emitter of methane in the US is the natural gas and petroleum industry (30 percent).

274. Dana Gunders, "Wasted: How America Is Losing Up to 40 Percent of Its Food from Farm to Fork to Landfill," issue brief no. 12-06-B, National Resources Defense Council, 2012.

275. "Mulch," *Organic Gardening*, http://www.organicgardening.com/learn-and-grow/mulch. Mulch is a gardening technique used to retain moisture in the soil, slow evaporation, and suppress weeds. Several materials can be used as mulch, including wood chips, newspaper, grass clippings, pebbles, etc.

"Where do you find your seeds?"

"I find organic seeds at grocery stores in the bulk bins. Rather than eat it, you plant it. And you can purchase them from organic seed companies found online."

"How do you manage your garden against pests?"

"Pests are part of nature. Hopefully, if a bad bug shows up, a good bug is right behind, or the robins and cardinals that nest in these trees are looking for a meal. I attract beneficial insects and birds into my garden by planting native trees and shrubs. If I have a pest infestation where the bugs can't be hand-picked, I make a homemade brew. I also use natural insecticides like Bt—*Bacillus thuringiensis*."[276]

Each year home gardeners pour sixty-four million pounds of pesticides (herbicides, insecticides and fungicides) on their gardens. While this represents only 16.7 percent of the total annual pesticide usage in the US, the amount has steadily increased over the last two decades.[277] Pesticides work to kill unwanted weeds and pests, but like on cropland, the chemicals inhibit the soil's ability to absorb water.[278]

2,4-D and glyphosate, the two most popular pesticides among home gardeners, are found in river and stream samples across the country.[279]

---

276. Bacillius thuringiensis (Bt) is a naturally occurring soil bacterium.

277. Arthur Grube et al., *Pesticides* "Industry Sales and Usage: 2006 and 2007 Market Estimates," US EPA, February 2011. https://www.epa.gov/pesticides.

278. Daniel Mada, Duniya N., and Idris G. Adams, "Effect of Continuous Application of Herbicide on Soil and Enviroment with Crop Protection Machinery in Southern Adamawa State," *International Refereed Journal of Engineering and Science* 2, no. 6 (June 2013), http://www.irjes.com/Papers/vol2-issue6/Version-2/B260409.pdf.

279. 2,4-D is found in 15 percent of rivers and streams sampled by the US Geological Survey (USGS). This total will increase with the approval of 2,4-D for use on genetically modified soy and corn in 2014. Glyphosate was detected in 32 percent of river and stream samples. It is higher in surface waters in the Midwest (40 percent), where there is a higher propensity of GM soy and corn fields. For information on glyphosate I referred to: RH Coupe, S.J. Kalkhoff, P.D. Capel, and C. Gregoire, "Fate and transport of glyphosate and aminomethylphosphonic acid in surface waters of agricultural basins," *Pesticide Management Science* 68 (2012): 16–30. For information on 2,4-D I referred to: Caroline Cox, "2,4-D," *Journal of Pesticide Reform* 25, no. 4 (2005): 10–15.

These pesticides favored in home gardens are the same as those applied on genetically modified corn and soy crops in the US and worldwide.

We make one last stop before we return to Manhattan: the Joe Holzka Community Garden in Staten Island.

"These provide shade and are rain harvesters," Lenny says while pointing out a shade structure with an inverted aluminum roof shining bright in the sunlight. "GrowNYC built these multi-purpose structures in community gardens around the city. Rain rolls down to the rain gutter along the center of the inverted roof. The water conveyed from the plastic pipes flows to the holding tank." We stand underneath the rain harvester, our hideaway from the sultry midday sun.

"Does this roof capture enough to water the garden?" The large parcel is crowded with raised beds, a buffer from the contaminated soil of the once-vacant lot.

"The holding tank waters a portion of this garden. The rest comes from the fire hydrant. In the winter, the tank is closed. Instead, the water is diverted into an underground pipe. All the water remains in the garden, no runoff into the city sewer system."

~

From the top deck of the Verrazano-Narrows Bridge on the return trip to Manhattan, water engulfs my vision in all directions. We move closer to the grand skyline. It seems to defy the laws of gravity with spires of concrete brushing against the clouds. If great cities like this one can be built, we can design gardens, yards, parks, and streets to harvest rainwater. I will start with my own garden.

Lenny's Homemade Pestaway Brew

Ingredients

1 spray bottle
1 tablespoon of organic liquid soap
2 crushed cloves of garlic
½ teaspoon of dried cayenne pepper
1 quart water

Directions

1. Mix ingredients together and pour into spray bottle.
2. Spray directly on the infected plants.
3. Repeat daily as needed.

Strawberry Rhubarb Crumble Pie

Makes 8 servings
30 minutes to prepare
35–45 minutes to bake

This is Kathy Venezia's, Lenny's wife and co-gardener, recipe for strawberry rhubarb pie. Rhubarb is a perennial vegetable. Buried under snow in the winter, it regrows in the spring. The hardy plant can regrow for several years. The tartness from the thick edible stalks of the plant is balanced with sweet strawberry in this springtime pie.

If you can't find rhubarb, swap with 1 cup celery and 1 cup chopped kale and reduce the sugar to ½ cup. This version is just as delicious.

Ingredients

FOR THE FILLING:

2 cups organic rhubarb stalks grown with rain-harvested water
2 cups organic strawberries
1 cup fair-trade organic sugar or local honey
2 teaspoons lemon zest
¼ cup organic lemon juice

FOR THE CRUMB TOPPING:

1 cup organic dry-farmed flour
¾ cup organic dried oats
4–6 ounces room-temperature, pasture-raised butter

½ cup fair-trade organic sugar or local honey
1 teaspoon lemon zest
dash of cinnamon

Directions

1. Preheat oven to 350°F.
2. Clean the rhubarb and cut into ½-inch pieces, rinse the strawberries and cut in half or quarters depending upon the size of the strawberries. If you want the flavors to blend, cut the fruit in thin slices although big, chunky pieces make a good pie too.
3. Mix rhubarb and strawberries in a bowl with sugar or honey.
4. Add lemon zest and about a ¼ cup of lemon juice and mix thoroughly.
5. In a separate bowl, mix the flour, oats, and butter for the crumb topping.
6. Add the remaining honey or sugar, lemon zest, and cinnamon.
7. Combine till they form small, little clumps.
8. Pour the rhubarb and strawberry mixture into a 9×12-inch greased glass pan. Form little dumplings with the dry mixture and cover the pan completely with the crumb topping.
9. Sprinkle a little sugar on the crumbs.
10. Bake for about 35–45 minutes. The pie is done when the liquid bubbles on the edge of the pan.

Grilled Vegetable Marinades

10 minutes to prepare

Grill time depends on vegetable thickness and variety

Lenny and his wife feast on the variety of vegetables they grow summer-long. With the subtle hint of herbs and olive oil and the sweet or savory flesh of fresh produce, grilled vegetables are the true show-stoppers of any meal. Grill times vary depending on the vegetable and the thickness. For example, zucchini sliced in ½-inch strips will grill in 3–5 minutes, but half an onion will take 30 minutes to grill. I slice vegetables the same thickness so they have similar cook times. A quick web search for vegetable grill times provides a helpful guide.

Here are their favorite marinades.

Lemon, Garlic, and Herb Marinade

Ingredients

1 cup dry-farmed olive oil
¾ cup of lemon or lime
2 cloves of crushed garlic
¼ cup freshly chopped herbs (ideas: parsley, cilantro, rosemary, thyme, or whatever you might have on hand)
salt and pepper to taste

Directions

1. Mix together ingredients in a bowl.
2. Prep your vegetables, cutting them in thick slices.
3. Soak the vegetables in the marinade or coat them with a brush.
4. Re-coat the vegetables as you grill for optimum flavor.

Caramelized Sweet and Sour Marinade

Ingredients

4 tablespoons of local honey
¼ cup dry-farmed olive oil
red pepper flakes to taste
juice from one orange (alternatively you can use 3 tablespoons of water)
¼ teaspoon salt

Directions

1. Mix ingredients in a blender or just shake them up in a covered bowl. Add some water if too dry.
2. Prep your vegetables, cutting them in thick slices. I especially like onions, sweet potatoes, and zucchini.
3. Soak the vegetables in the marinade or coat with a brush.
4. Re-coat the vegetables as you grill for optimum flavor.

Lemon Mint Marinade for Eggplant

Ingredients

¼ cup dry-farmed olive oil
¼ cup organic lemon juice
1 small bunch chopped fresh organic mint
salt to taste

Directions

1. Mix together ingredients in a bowl.
2. Slice eggplant horizontally into roughly ½-inch slices.
3. Brush the marinade on the eggplant as it grills.
4. Grill 5 minutes per side.

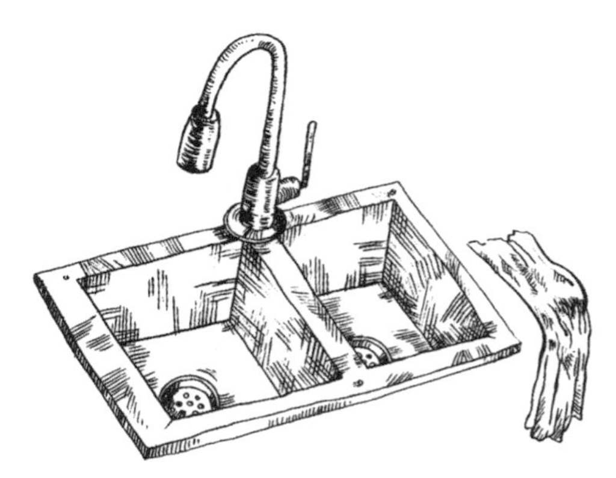

EPILOGUE

The Solution Is in the Kitchen

ON MARCH 22, Estrella, my youngest, stood next to my bed. When I opened my eyes, she handed me a homemade card and said, "Congratulations! Today is your day." On the front of the card, she drew the earth in a shape of a water drop with crayon. Inside, it read *Happy World Water Day.*

World Water Day was established in 1992 by the United Nations, to raise awareness of water issues and encourage action. More than twenty-five years later, the international day of observance passes largely unnoticed.

When the well is dry, we know the value of water, wrote Benjamin Franklin. For 800 million people around the world, the well has gone dry. For three long years, the well was dry for 1,500 families in California's San Joaquin Valley, the "food basket of the world." Many of these families, many of whom work on irrigated fields of crops exported around the world, spent up to 10 percent of their income to purchase bottled water for drinking and bathing.[280] For the 98,310 residents of Flint, Michigan, water runs from the taps but is too dirty to drink. The water from Flint

280. Community Water Center, http://www.communitywatercenter.org/challenge.

River, polluted from industry, landfills, and agricultural fields upstream, is tainted with heavy metals and harmful bacteria (E. coli, coliform from fecal matter).[281] Water scarcity has become a way of life for indigenous communities in Alaska, with their water source contaminated from run-off from long-abandoned mines.

Water experts predict the situation will worsen, with two-thirds of the world's population predicted to be without a clean, reliable source of water within a quarter century.

This book in many ways is my version of a homemade card written to celebrate and bring awareness to water. But it's not "your day," as Estrella wrote in her Earth Day card, it is *our* day. The problem of water scarcity doesn't belong only to those whose glass is empty. Water belongs to us collectively.

The farmers and food producers I present in this book illustrate the very *best* in food cultivation. This food is grown with farming systems in sync with the surrounding environment, working to replenish rivers, not pollute them. They represent farming methods that regenerate the soil, thereby keeping more water in the ground so the well never goes dry.

According to a 2015 Gallup Poll, 44 percent of Americans "include organic" in their food purchases. But what the poll doesn't ask is "How often?" In the same year, 3 percent of food produced and sold in the United States was grown without chemicals, antibiotics, petroleum-based fertilizers, or genetically modified seeds designed to be paired with pesticides. If 44 percent of eaters "include organic," why are we not supporting more organic agriculture? Three percent is not enough to reverse the damage of pollution from agriculture on our rivers, lakes, and oceans. And it falls

281. Joseph M. Leonardi and William J. Gruhn, "Alaska Department of Natural Resources 2001 Annual Report," State of Michigan D epartment of Natural Resources 27 (2001), http://www.michigandnr.com/PUBLICATIONS/PDFS/ifr/ifrlibra/Special/Reports/sr27.pdf; "Flint Water Crisis," *CNN*, August 2016, http://www.cnn.com/2016/03/04/us/flint-water-crisis-fast-facts.

short in halting the practice of drawing down groundwater resources to irrigate thirsty crop fields treated with chemicals.[282]

"How wonderful, the work those farmers are doing," people often tell me. "It is admirable work," they say. I agree with them. With all my heart I agree. But this small army of sustainable farmers, fishermen, ranchers, and food and beverage producers need more than our admiration; they need our business. Saving water is a team effort. It is us, the *eaters*, who propagate, cultivate, and nourish farmers/food producers to produce the *best* food for water so they can "keep doing how we do," as Kristan Fretwell from Hunter Cattle says.

A year after my visit to Kurt Unkel's rice fields, he closed his farm business, Cajun Grain. Too few people took the time and energy to find his rice that uses 40 percent less water than the average flooded rice paddy. He refused rice subsidies, and instead worked toward a vision of farming the land for improved nutrition. When I was on his farm in Louisiana, he tenderly held a rice plant in his hand and spoke of his commitment to building healthy soil. "If the soil is healthy, the plant is healthy, and we are healthy," he told me. As much as it broke his heart, he could no longer afford to wait for the *eater*.

Rick Goche, an albacore fisherman in Oregon coastal waters, explained to me how salmon travel hundreds of miles upstream to return to the water of their birth. The arduous journey of the salmon is made more difficult and sometimes impossible by the damming of rivers. Small-scale family farms in our modern agricultural system are like salmon swimming against the current tide.

Darinka and Paul Postal raised a small flock of pasture-raised organic chickens between the trees of an orange orchard in Ojai Valley, California. Their farms generated zero waste. The chicken manure on their farm fertilized the orchard, and not a single chicken was wasted; instead slaughter totals matched the number of orders. Darinka and

282. This total doesn't include those farmers who practice "organic" farming (no chemicals, no petroleum-based fertilizers) but are not certified, but their numbers are too small to make an impact on this statistic.

Paul closed down their farm operation because they weren't selling enough chickens to be profitable. They needed to sell at the farmers' market, but because they processed in the open air, regulations kept them from selling their meat at the farmers' market or the local butcher. They were too small to succeed.

At Hunter Cattle, located an hour outside Savannah, Georgia, the mobile chicken boxes, like the ones used at Funny Farms, were empty. When I asked about it, Kristan Fretwell told me that legally they can process up to 1,000 chickens in the open air. She described how the whole family pitched in to process chickens: children, nephews, and spouses. "The day we processed chickens was one of my favorite days," she said. "We sold the chickens in our store on the premises, and the chicken always sold out. The fields are better when we have chickens. We moved the mobile houses behind the cattle. The birds ate all the bugs and spread the food for us."

"Why did you stop?" I asked her.

"The USDA inspector is in-house five days a week and said they preferred we stop processing chickens outside since we have a processing facility for beef, pork, and lamb even though we didn't break any rules. She didn't want any cross-contamination, so we stopped processing chickens. And because the closest chicken processing place requires a minimum of 400 birds to process and is four hours away, we stopped raising chickens altogether."

During my visit with Kristan, she explained to me how food and safety regulations are designed for the "big dogs" as she calls them, large agricultural operations that dominate every food group in America. For example, with each grind of ground beef, an E.coli test is required. "Of course, that's an important test," said Kristan. "But we might have one to two cows in each grind and each test costs one hundred dollars. The *big dogs* will have a grind of hundreds if not thousands of cows in one grind and still only need the one test." The one-size-fits-all approach to food regulations works against small farms.

Since my visit to Benziger Family Winery in Northern California, the winery was sold to the third largest wine company in the world by volume. The sale is indicative of the market consolidation of food production. The newer corporate owner pledged to preserve the "green farming" practices cultivated for over three decades. According to Mike Benziger, the technologies employed on the farm influenced the purchase. Time will tell if the practices from the winery will influence the corporation's overall operations. Regardless of whether the new owners of Benziger will *water down* the conservation efforts implemented under the tutelage of Mike Benziger and his family, or seize the opportunity to deepen what they began, the blueprint for the *best* way to grow wine grapes remains.

In the beginning of this book, I describe a conversation I had with my eldest child in the kitchen. My daughter asked why the cupboards had only organic cereal. My answer, *because it is better for water* is when I began to put food into categories of *better* and *best*. It guides my food choices. But I don't always eat and serve the best foods. I cook, serve, eat a mixture of better and best foods for water, and sometimes the worst foods. Everything in life is a work in progress. Each time we make a decision to eat less water, it is like tossing a pebble into still water, causing a ripple effect.

The *best* foods for water:

1. Are grown without petroleum fertilizers and pesticides.
2. Are grown or raised with *green* water like dry-farmed and rain-fed foods.
3. Use water-efficient irrigation like drip irrigation, water catchment, and closed-loop systems.

4. Are meat and animal products raised on pasture-based operations. Ruminant animals and poultry (including egg-layers) are from farms where the animals are rotationally grazed (e.g., holistic-managed, mob-grazed, managed intentional rotational grazing).
5. Are from animal operations that use no hormones or antibiotics in feed.
6. Are grown on small-scale, diverse farm operations.
7. Are wild-caught seafood with sustainable fishing methods like pole and line and trolling from regulated fisheries, like those in the United States.

The *best* action steps to institute in our kitchens for water are:

1. Waste less food by planning meals and keeping perishable foods front and center in the refrigerator (30–50 percent of all food is thrown away).
2. Buy fewer meat and dairy products (the average American eats 270 pounds of meat, 250 eggs, and 630 pounds of dairy each year).
3. Support local sustainable agriculture and shop at a farmers' market.
4. Cook meals from scratch as much as possible to control the source of your ingredients (when you eat out, follow the same rules for *best* food).
5. Teach the children in your life how to cook and why food choices matter to the health of our environment. My three young children each choose, plan, and cook a meal a week. They were handed knives at a young age. My hope is when they graduate to their own kitchens they will continue to implement the practices they learned in mine. The next generation of *eaters* needs to be active participants if we are to fundamentally change food systems. Compost food waste (decomposition of food waste in landfills and wastewater treatment plants accounts for 20 percent of methane emissions).

We can influence change. A survey among top corporations found *customers* to be the leading driver of their company's sustainability initiatives. Customers are over two times more influential to sustainability decisions than company shareholders and three times more than policy-holders and non-governmental organizations.[283] Larger companies are taking notice of the growing American preference for organic foods.[284]

We hold the power to change the way food is grown and produced in the United States: we the eaters.

There is power in the collective, I write at the end of each of my blog posts. It is the idea that gives me hope. We can influence food systems to grow and produce our food differently, but only if we merge our influence. "It's a combination of all these little things that will fix things," said Kurt Unkel. He plans to return to farming. Collectively we will rewrite the story of the future of water on this exquisite planet we call home.

---

283. "Six Growing Trends in Corporate Sustainability: Employees Emerge as a Key Stakeholder Group for Sustainability Programs and Reporting," Ernst & Young, http://www.ey.com/US/en/Services/Specialty-Services/Climate-Change-and-Sustainability-Services/Six-growing-trends-in-corporate-sustainability_Trend-3.

284. This also includes natural foods. There is no definition of "natural" food. I tend to stay clear of natural foods as I find the ingredients to include palm oil, GMOs (unless otherwise noted on the box), and high corn fructose syrup. Conversely, organic foods must follow strict guidelines for the certification.

Index of Recipes

Joaquin's Favorite Homemade Pasta 22

Mama's Whole Wheat Bread 25

Cajun Grain's Brown Rice Pancakes 42

Nelida's Cheese, Swiss Chard,
and Kale Tamales 53

Tofu over Sautéed Asian Greens 64

Pole and Line or Troll-Caught Tuna and
Organic Gorgonzola Quesadillas 77

Wild-Caught Baked Salmon 79

Carney's Country Style Grits 86

Green Eggs, Asparagus,
and Spinach Quiche 96

Funny Farm's Simple Roasted Chicken
and Seasonal Vegetables 103

Next-Night Chicken Tortilla Soup 105

Cobblestone Farm's Crustless Cheesecake
with Fresh Strawberry Topping 121

Managed Intensive Rotationally Grazed,
Pasture-Raised Grilled Burgers
with Homemade Organic Buns 138

Homemade Organic Buns.................. 141

Taza Hot Chocolate........................ 155

Taza Chocolate Mexicano Cookies........... 157

How to Brew the Best Cup of Coffee......... 169

Alquimia-rita.............................. 189

Michael's Organic Dark Ale Two-Bean Chili
with Beef or Tempeh.................... 200

Greenstar Spent Grain Burgers.............. 203

Lenny's Homemade Pestaway Brew.......... 215

Strawberry Rhubarb Crumble Pie............ 216

Grilled Vegetable Marinades................ 218

IN GRATITUDE

Writing a book is a lot like baking bread. It takes time, patience, and faith to transform the flour, water, and yeast from a sticky mess into one smooth mound of dough ready to rise.

First and foremost, thanks be to God for trusting to me write this book.

Thank you to the fierce and brilliant women writers in my life. Especially to the members of my writing group: Mona Alvarado, Lori Braun, Danielle Brown, Toni Guy, Amada Irma Perez, and Sheri Ward. They've read and re-read these pages, offering me guidance, feedback, and urging me forward. Special thanks to A Room of Her Own Foundation (AROHO) for awarding me the Gift of Freedom in Creative Non-Fiction. The prize came with a cash gift, invaluable life-coaching sessions from author Gail McMeekin, and the priceless validation that *Eat Less Water*, still in its infancy, needed to be written. In gratitude, to Darlene Chandler Bassett, co-founder of AROHO, who walked with me on this journey that was both scenic and arduous.

Thank you to Kate Gale, managing editor of Red Hen Press, for loving this book after a shot of the "Tequila & Water" chapter. I am proud to publish with this indie press committed to printing diverse voices and to work with Red Hen's small and mighty staff.

A special thanks to editor extraordinaire, Dennis Mathis from Close Readers Group. He is worth his weight in gold, but thankfully accepted much, much less because he believed in the importance of this book.

In gratitude to the farmers and food and beverage producers who answered my call—literally. Each of them are the heroes of this story, working daily to protect our soil, air, and water. Thank you to Darinka and Paul Postal, my very first hosts. Darinka was first a teacher to my children, then my teacher of sustainable farming. To John DeRosier, I'll never forget our first phone conversation. When I explained to him the premise for my book, he said, "You are in for a treat." I was served a chocolate cake that day. Thank you to Dr. Adolfo Murillo for inviting me into his dining room in Oxnard and patiently walking me through the science of distillation (and for the bottle of tequila). Thanks to Mike Benziger for championing biodynamics on California vineyards.

Thank you to Alex Whitman, who makes the lives of Latin American cacao farmers sweeter with the production of Taza chocolate. Thank you to Lenny Librizzi for inviting me into his Staten Island garden, and for his work collecting rain in the five Burroughs of New York. Special thanks to Maureen and Paul Knapp, for opening my eyes to holistic management and the art of grazing animals. It changed the way I approached every farm thereafter.

Thank you to Alfred and Carney Farris, two pioneers in the sustainable farming movement, building their Tennessee soil for fifty years with wisdom and grace. I will never forget my time with Kurt Unkel. Instead of water, he floods his rice fields with passion. Thank you to Ben Godfrey for showing me how aquaculture can support sustainable agriculture. Rob Cunningham made a lasting impression on me, not because he is the tallest man I've ever met, or because of his jealous cow Jolene, but for proving that producing organic, pastured eggs on a rotational system is feasible on a larger scale.

A special thanks to Kristan Fretwell and her vibrant family. I will retell many of the stories she told me that didn't make this book but are too good not to tell. Thank you to Hillery and Erik Gunther for letting me walk in the clouds with them one winter morning. They've taken the adage "Leave things better than when you found them" to a whole new level.

Profound gratitude to Nelida Martinez; her life is an embodiment of Maya Angelou's words *But still, like dust, I'll rise.* From Nelida's dust rises chemical-free vegetables for her family and community.

Rick Goche unknowingly took the task of explaining sustainable seafood to me in a handful of hours. He succeeded by being who he is and generously imparting his experience that stretches decades and thousand of nautical miles.

Helen and Mike Cameron's restaurant Uncommon Ground and Greenstar Brewery takes the farm-to-table concept through the roof with their certified organic rooftop farm. Special thanks to Martin Coad for walking me through the organic and conventional beer-making process.

Several years ago, I sat in a statistics study group. I looked at the board scribbled with math notations and thought, *I'm glad I don't need to pay attention to this*. My mind snapped back into attention with the recognition that my exam was the following day. This is my convoluted way of thanking the Irving B. Harris School of Public Policy. Without those math courses, I couldn't have written this book. It was at the University of Chicago where I met some of the smartest people I've ever met. I am especially thankful to the members of the inaugural Minorities in Public Policy Studies Club (MIPPS). I couldn't have survived economic derivates without them.

A heartfelt thank you to my mom and pa. They taught me by example to feel compassion for the people and the world around me. From my mother, I learned to be a teacher and from my father, to be an activist; it is this blend that gave birth to this book.

Isabella, Joaquin, and Estrella, now ten, eleven, and fourteen, walked this journey with me. They sacrificed while I was in the kitchen kneading this bread. I thank them for their patience, understanding, and unconditional love. Each of them inspired this work. I refuse to leave them a water-scarce world without a fight. I love them too much.

To my husband Michael; without him, there is no book. He recognized this project was my *path with a heart* and did everything to clear away the thick brush. It's unimaginable to love a man more. Anything is possible with his love, like writing a book about water. All paths lead to Michael, *para siempre*.

To the reader, thank you for opening your heart and mind to the concepts presented in this book. Let us break bread and change the world together.

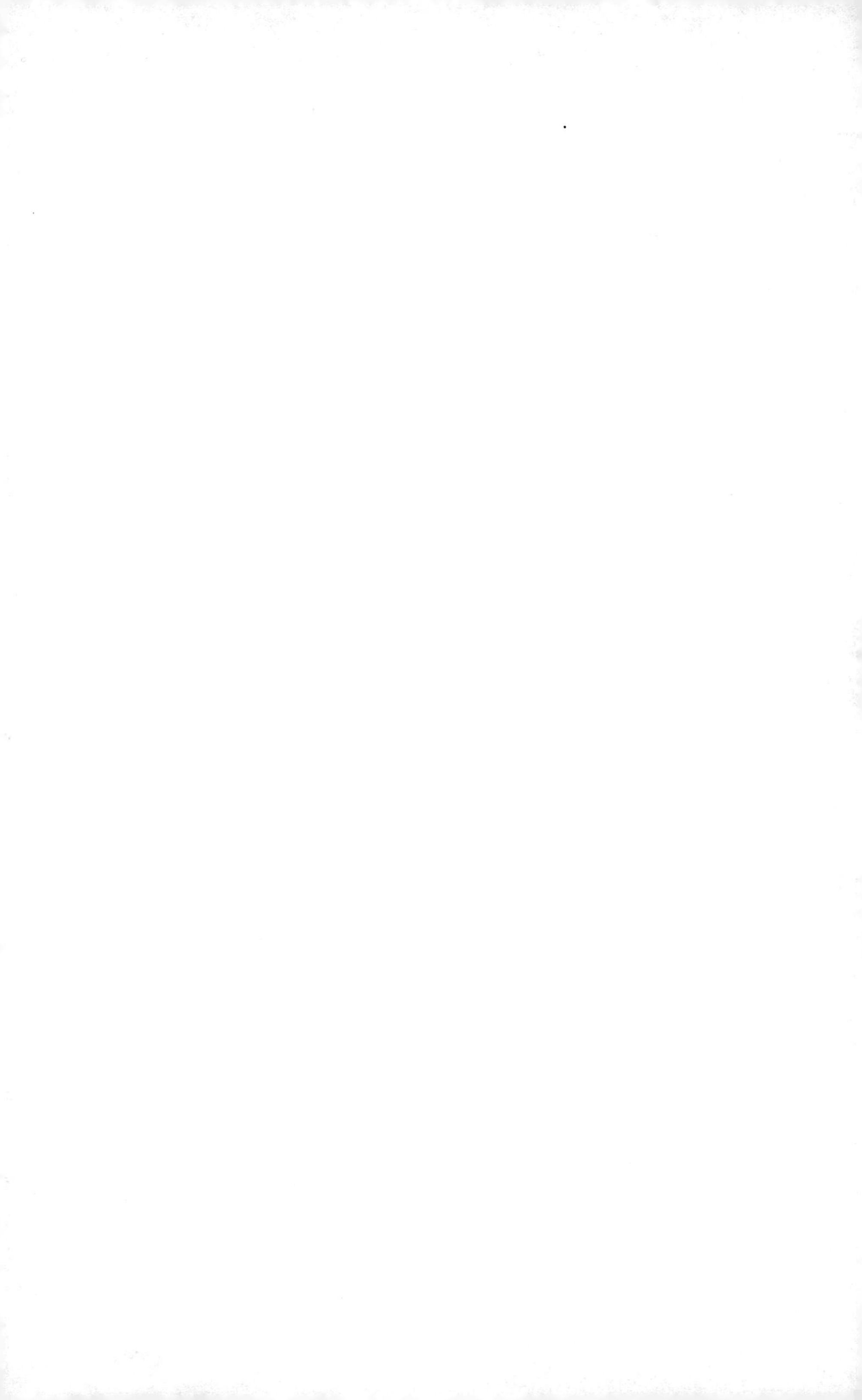

BIOGRAPHICAL NOTE

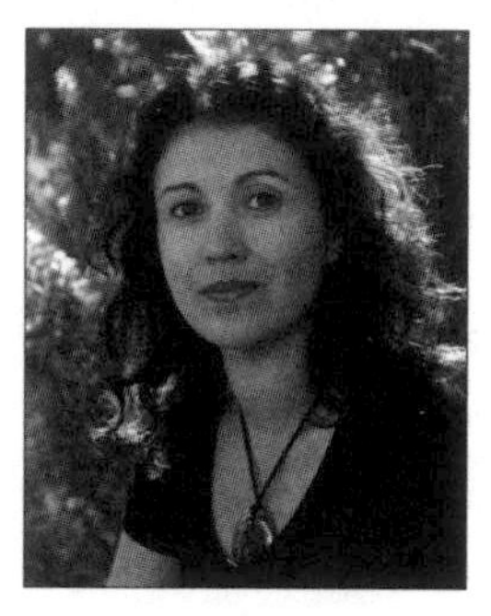

Florencia Ramirez is a researcher trained at the University of Chicago's Harris School of Public Policy. She won the sixth Gift of Freedom Creative Nonfiction Award from the A Room of Her Own Foundation (AROHO). Her articles appear in *Edible Communities Magazine*, the *San Jose Mercury News*, among others, and in her popular blog. She lives in Oxnard, California, an agricultural town on the Pacific coast that smells of celery, strawberries, and fertilizers with her husband and three young children. Visit her website at www.florenciaramirez.com.